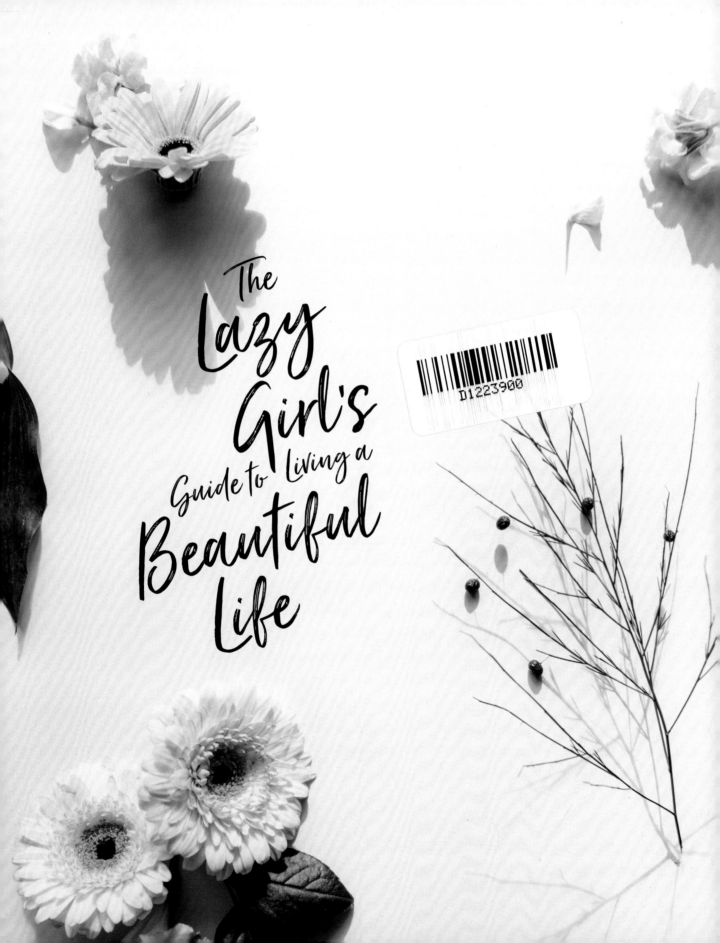

The Lazy Girl's Guide to Living a Beautiful Life

D1223900

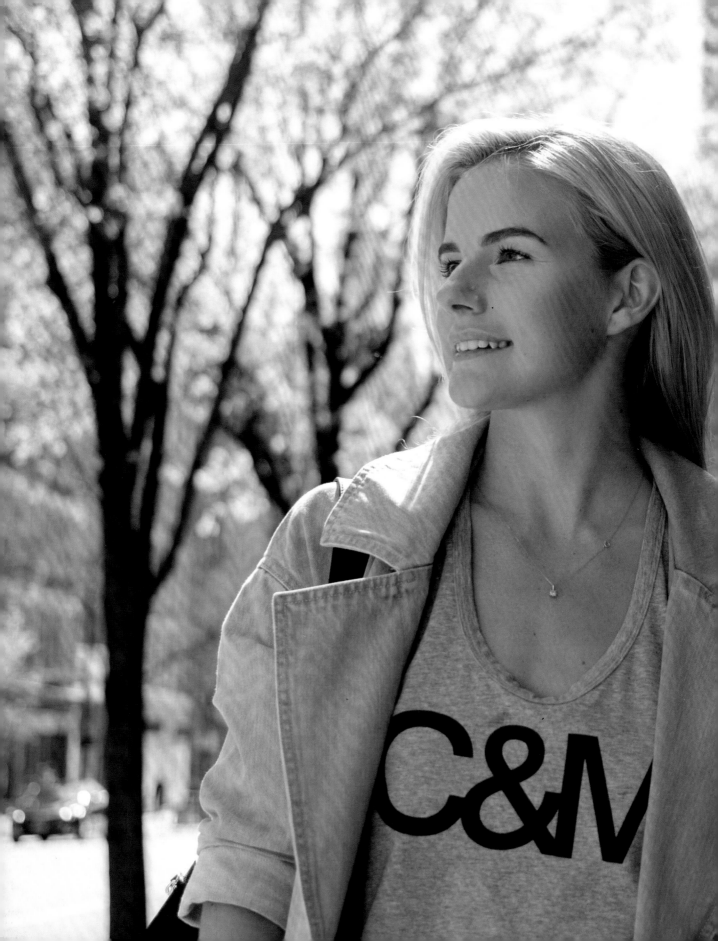

The Lazy Girl's Guide to Living a Beautiful Life

MATILDA RICE

ALLEN&UNWIN

SYDNEY • MELBOURNE • AUCKLAND • LONDON

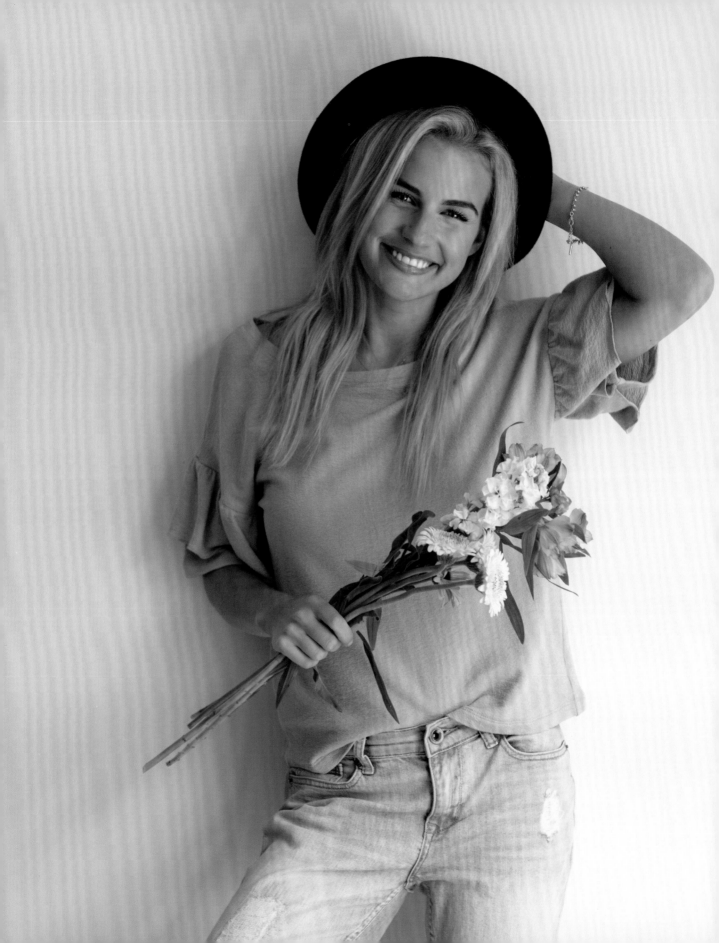

CONTENTS

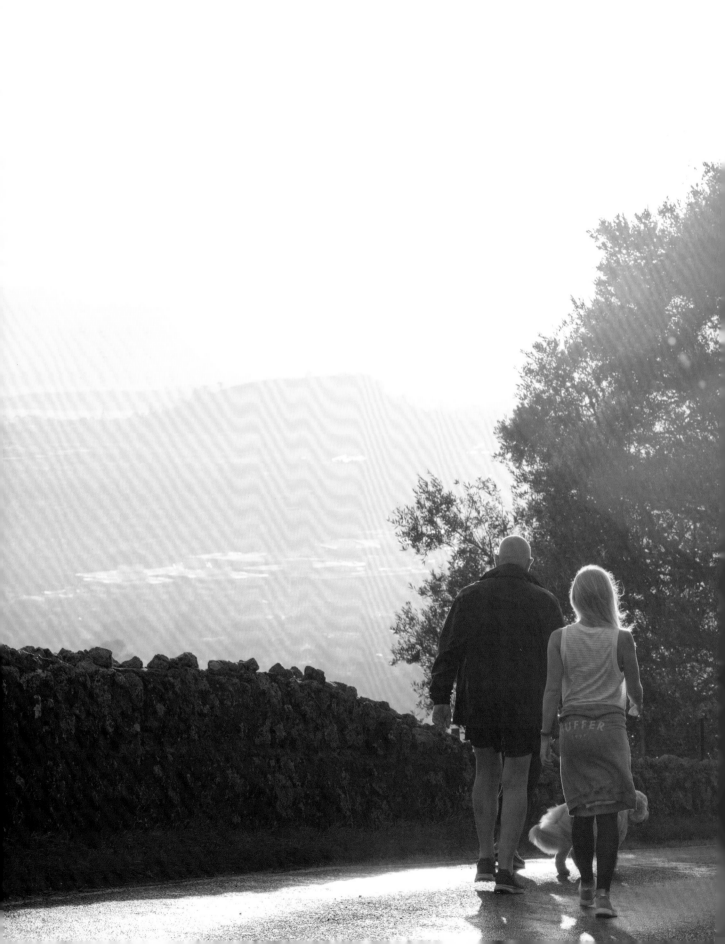

FOREWORD

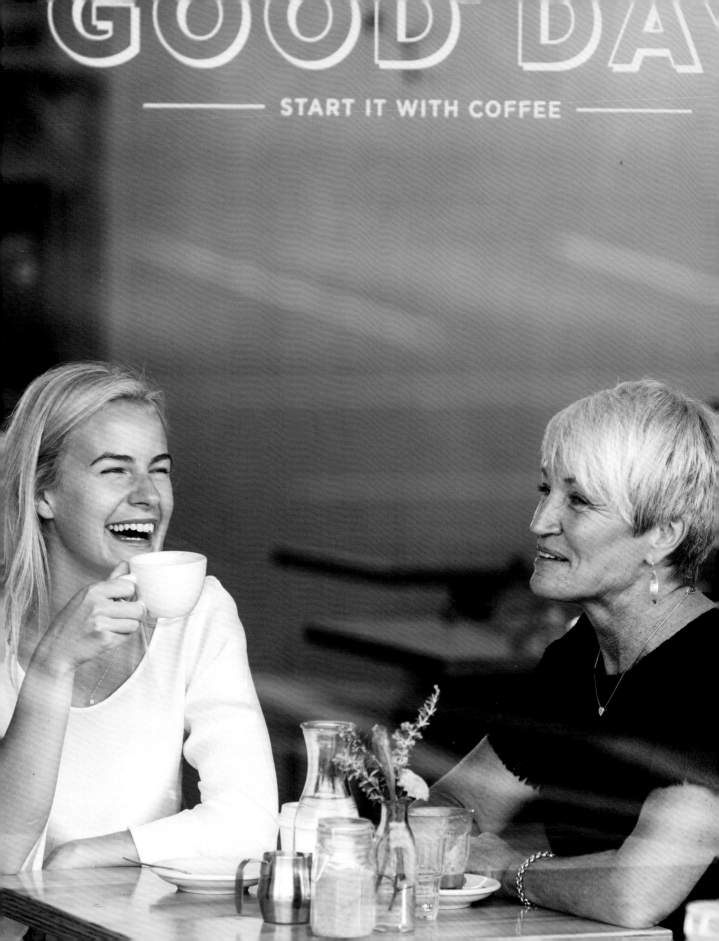

A NOTE FROM
MATILDA'S MUM

––––––––––

Firstly, I should point out that, since I'm Matilda's mother, you'll have to remember that my views may not be 100 per cent objective or unbiased! But, I have obviously known Matilda all her life, and watched her progress from infancy through childhood, her teenage years and young adulthood, to becoming the wonderful young woman she is today. So, what I *can* do is provide a context for the journey that has resulted in this book that you hold in your hands.

Like many little people, Matilda had a 'difficult' relationship with food when she was growing up. Around the age of two, she developed an extremely strong aversion to any form of fruit or vegetable. She had a finely tuned antenna for detecting anything green on her plate, no matter how expertly or creatively I tried to camouflage it. Every time, discovery led to a very firm (but very polite) 'No thank you' from Matilda. Fruit was even worse; the wet and slimy textures would make her physically gag. Many of you are already familiar with her love of mince, and I can attest to the fact that that particular love affair began way back then. She survived her entire childhood almost exclusively on spag bol and whole milk! How she managed to evade the ravages of scurvy was a mystery to her concerned grandmothers, godmothers and aunties for many, many years.

Food, to me, has always been about love, nurturing and social enjoyment, so I never wanted dinner time to be a battleground. We just made sure we always had lots of back-up spag bol in the freezer. I did often joke that I thought Matilda would grow up to be a vegetarian, as her body's way of compensating for the lack of fruit and veges in her childhood—and, as it turned out, I was almost right on the money!

Matilda's discovery of a healthy and balanced lifestyle has been her own journey.

It has been a journey influenced by her travels, by her peers, by her family and by her happiness. The years of living in flats with nothing much in the fridge and weeks' worth of fast-food wrappers in her car, while partying hard and sleeping late, were pretty much a rite of passage. Sport and exercise were never much of a priority, either. I seem to remember Matilda managed to get through one whole school year without finding her 'lost' P.E. gear, thus avoiding the dreaded compulsory sport as much as possible.

It was while living in London that Matilda eventually discovered exercise—and fruit! She might not be a natural athlete, but has enormous determination when she decides to undertake a project. Her wonderful humour and ability to enjoy life to the max (while not taking it too seriously) have finally seen her get the food/exercise/living/relaxation/fun equation pretty balanced.

I couldn't be prouder.

Di Rice
November 2017

A NOTE FROM MATILDA'S DAD

I first met Matilda at about 4 a.m. on Monday, 22 October 1990. She was looking a little the worse for wear, but I guess that was to be expected—she had, after all, just been born! She was a very welcome addition to our family, and little were we to know the impact she would have on our lives or indeed on the lives of all those around her.

As time went on and Matilda grew, it became clear that she had been born with a mind of her own. Obstinate? Pigheaded? Nope, none of that. Matilda was *resolute*! She knew her own mind from day one. It surprised me every now and then over the years, but I came to have complete faith in her life decisions, and if I ever did find myself questioning things I knew that Matilda would have the resolve to right herself—and she always did.

It was a great ambition of Matilda's mum and me to get Matilda to eat her fruit and vegetables. So imagine our surprise when, picking her up from kindy one day, we were informed by Maree the Cook (there was also a Maree the Boss, you see) that Matilda just *loved* her vegetable quiche. Cut to the dinner conversation that night:

'So, Matilda, we learned today how much you love vegetable quiche at kindy. Care to explain?'

'That's at *kindy*, Dad!'

What happened at kindy stayed at kindy, apparently.

Matty didn't like school; she couldn't see the point, really. Upon leaving school, she travelled, gained marvellous life experiences, fell on her face a few times, picked herself up, dusted herself off and carried on, convinced that she would eventually find her niche, her happiness, her love and—oh, parental joy of joys!—fruit and vegetables. (Matilda has even included a recipe of mine that she's called the 'best roast veges you'll ever eat', should you care to go to that page first. Just sayin'!)

And that resolve I mentioned earlier? Well, that has shown up in so many ways with Matilda. This book is a prime example. Matilda had no doubt that she could write it, no doubt that it would be something people would want to read, and is in no doubt that it will be of great benefit to you, dear reader, should you wish to achieve even a modicum of health and happiness.

Enjoy your copy.

Read it and use it as many times as you can.

Matilda wrote it especially for you, with love—and with great resolve!

Ken Rice
November 2017

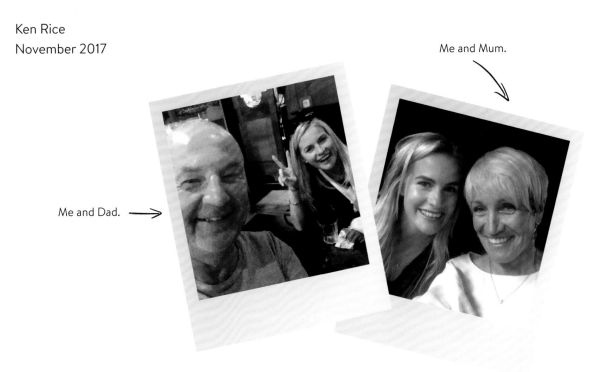

Me and Mum.

Me and Dad.

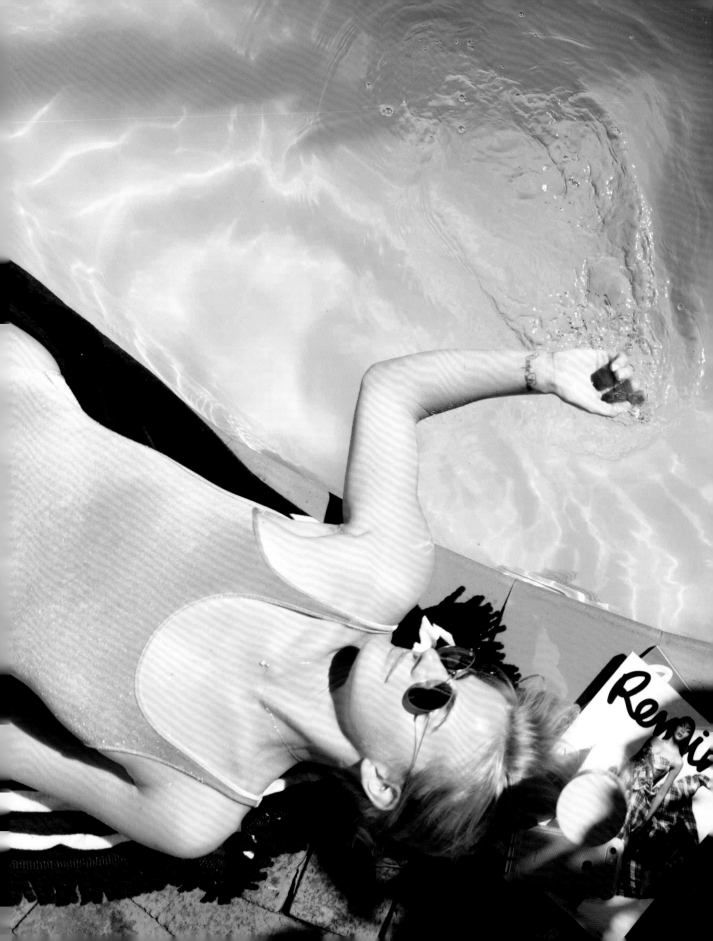

INTRODUCTION

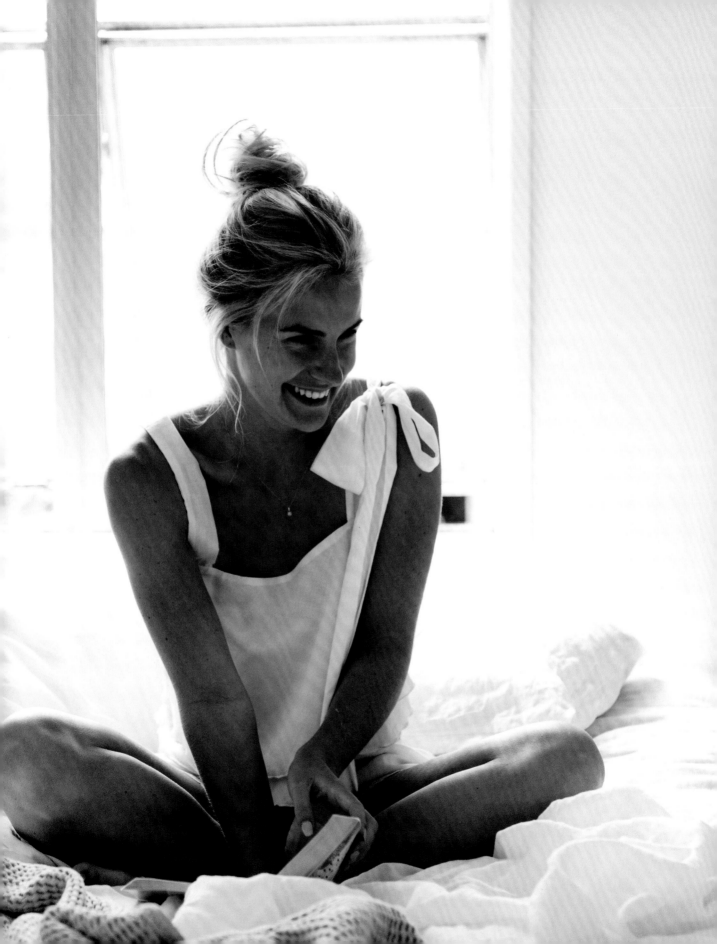

Hi! If you've picked up this book, chances are that you:
a) are also lazy
b) want to live a more positive, balanced life through health and wellness
c) both of the above, or
d) you can't speak English so were drawn in by the pretty pictures and
therefore you're not reading this at all . . .

If you answered 'c) both of the above', you're in the same boat I was in. I am naturally incredibly lazy and disorganised. It's one of those annoying traits I feel like you're born with, and for ages I thought that was just how I was wired and there was nothing I could do about it. Being unproductive (or just straight-up lazy, let's be honest) was simply how I would have to live my life, I thought, and I'd resigned myself to that fact. I wasn't even really that bothered about it.

The thing is, I have so many friends who fall into the 'doer' category. Ugh, doers are the *worst*! Always being productive and crossing things off lists and stuff . . . I hate those people. Jokes, I love them really. Plus, where would the world be without doers? There would be nothing!

There was no way I could ever become a doer—or so I thought. Well, fellow lazy friends, I have good news for all of us: it's possible to be both a lazy girl *and* a doer! Or, at least just enough of a doer to find your way to a happy, fun, healthy and productive life. A beautiful life! I know, because I've done it, and am living proof. The beauty of it is that I'm not asking you to completely abandon your lazy tendencies (I certainly haven't), and I'm not asking you to make any extreme lifestyle changes. Who can be bothered with that? Instead, it's about embracing and recognising everything that is already awesome about yourself—including your chilled approach to life—at the same time as creating some great new habits to help your life be even better. It's not even hard work.

According to the Myers-Briggs personality test, I'm an ESFJ personality type. That stands for Extravert, Sensing, Feeling, Judging, and means I've got great traits like being empathetic and caring . . . but also that I'm not so good with productivity. These days,

The Myers-Briggs Personality Test

The Myers-Briggs test is a popular personality test that sorts personalities into sixteen different types based on four fundamental psychological functions: sensation, intuition, feeling and thinking. The test was developed by Isabel Briggs Myers and her mother, Katherine Briggs, and identifies different personality types based on how each of us react to different situations—for example, whether we tend to respond to things rationally or perceptively.

The test gives you a personality 'type' that is a four-letter combination of the following character traits:

Extraversion (E) or **Introversion (I)**
Sensing (S) or **Intuition (N)**
Thinking (T) or **Feeling (F)**
Judging (J) or **Perceiving (P)**

It sounds more complicated than it actually is, and it often nails aspects of your behaviour that you didn't even notice until they're pointed out to you! If nothing else, it's fun to do with your friends or family. You can find lots of places online to do the test for free, and more information here: www.myersbriggs.org.

though, I feel like I've managed to hit the sweet spot where I have the bare minimum of 'doing' in my life, but just enough that I also have a healthy body and mind, a good level of fitness and overall happiness. The great thing about hitting that sweet spot is that once you start to feel healthier and happier your goals start to get bigger, and you begin to introduce even more good habits—and that all flows into every aspect of your life. It's a win-win!

These days, I'm more of a doer than ever before. This has stemmed from a few different things. In my life post-*The Bachelor* I found that I was increasingly time-poor from having so many different things on the go all at once, and this forced me to take a look at my productivity levels (or lack thereof) and figure out where I needed to make changes for the sake of my peace of mind. I *hate* it when you feel like life is on top of you, and like you can't get your head above water, so these days I make sure to avoid that feeling by writing absolutely everything I need to do down and being smarter with my time.

I also think, as I've got older, I've come to realise that I need to become a little bit more of a doer. I started to notice that problems don't just go away if you ignore them. (I know—who knew?!) Being an adult with responsibilities forced me to organise my life simply to make it easier. I now love spreadsheets! I never thought I would say such a thing, but they are just the best.

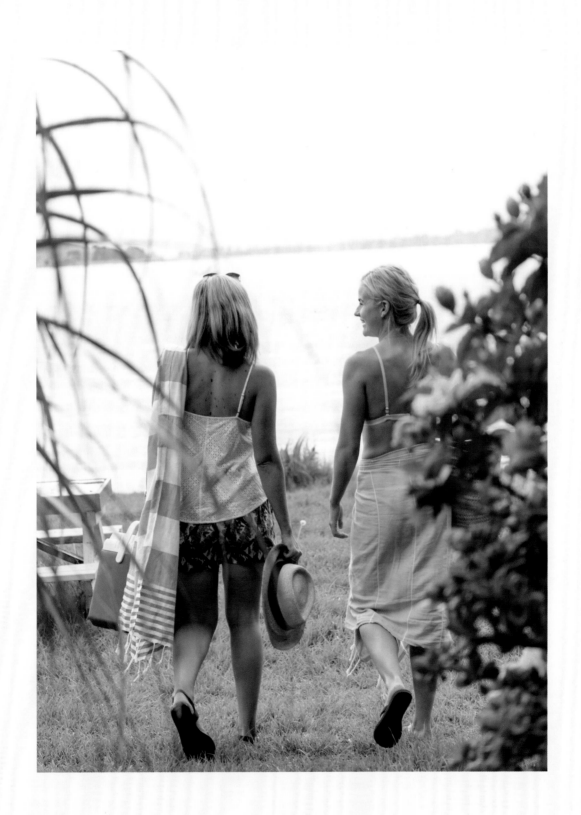

———

I'M A HUGE
ADVOCATE OF
SELF-LOVE AND OF
LISTENING TO YOUR
BODY, WHICH IS
ALWAYS TELLING
YOU SOMETHING.

———

So here I am: a lazy girl who's also a bit of a doer!

I've found that the process of learning to look after myself from the inside has positively transferred to so much on the outside. Nowadays I'm fitter than I've ever been, have a more positive outlook on things, have developed some great ways of dealing with stress, and am far more productive than ever before. Plus, I feel pretty great about who I am as a person. It's important when you say something like that to genuinely believe it—and if you don't yet, then I hope this book can help to convince you!

I'm a huge advocate of self-love and of listening to your body, which is *always* telling you something. It's not as easy as it sounds to practise self-love and to get in the habit of hearing what your body's saying to you. It's not something you wake up one day and decide to do and then that's it: self-love sorted! It's an ongoing process, and something that you have to work at every day. I'm yet to meet anyone who has fully mastered either of these things just yet.

And you know what? We can be so hard on our poor bodies sometimes. *Why aren't you skinny enough? Why can't you run faster or for longer? Why will that cellulite not GO AWAY?!* I'm sure a few of you might have asked yourselves one or two of these common questions at some point or another. But let me ask you this: how would you react if someone said those things to you? I certainly wouldn't be happy about it. In fact, if someone asked me any one of those questions, I probably wouldn't like that person very much at all. I imagine your body probably feels the same way when you are constantly mean to it. Our bodies deserve better than that. They work so hard for us every day— breathing, moving about, fighting anything they deem detrimental to us—and we hardly ever think to be thankful to our bodies for everything they quietly do. They just work away behind the scenes, doing everything they can to keep you healthy. It's OK to be nice to your body. In fact, it's quite important.

I hope this book will inspire you not only to look and feel your best, but also to treat yourself and your body as your best friend, because that's how things should be. If you're a bit of a lazy girl like me, I hope it will also help you to embrace just enough of the doer side of yourself to live the best life you can. And, if nothing else, I hope you maybe get a laugh out of one of my stories. Trust me, there are some real nuggets in here.

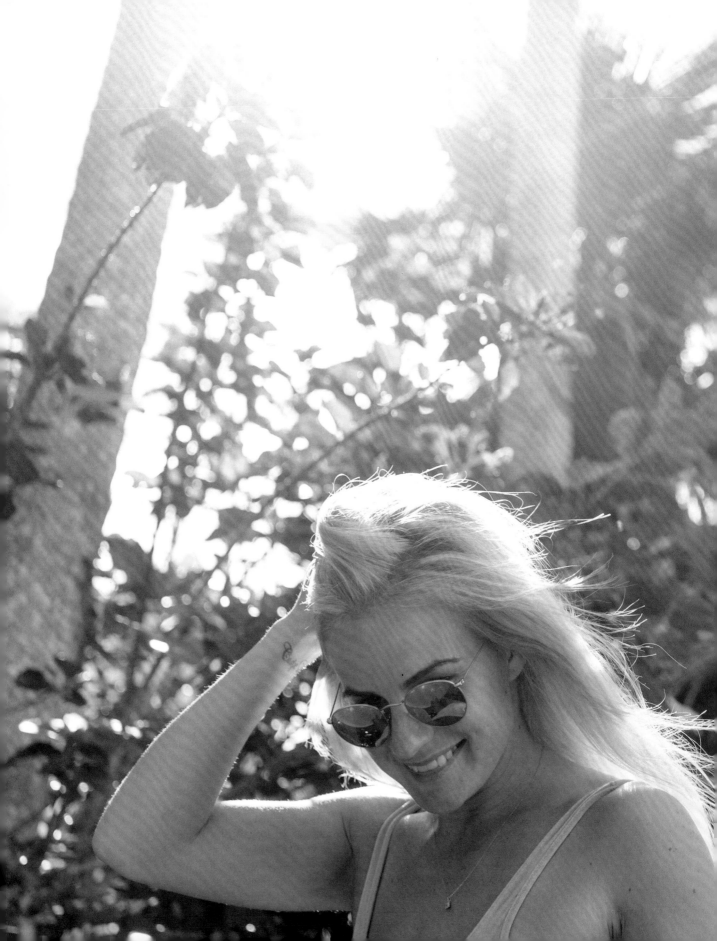

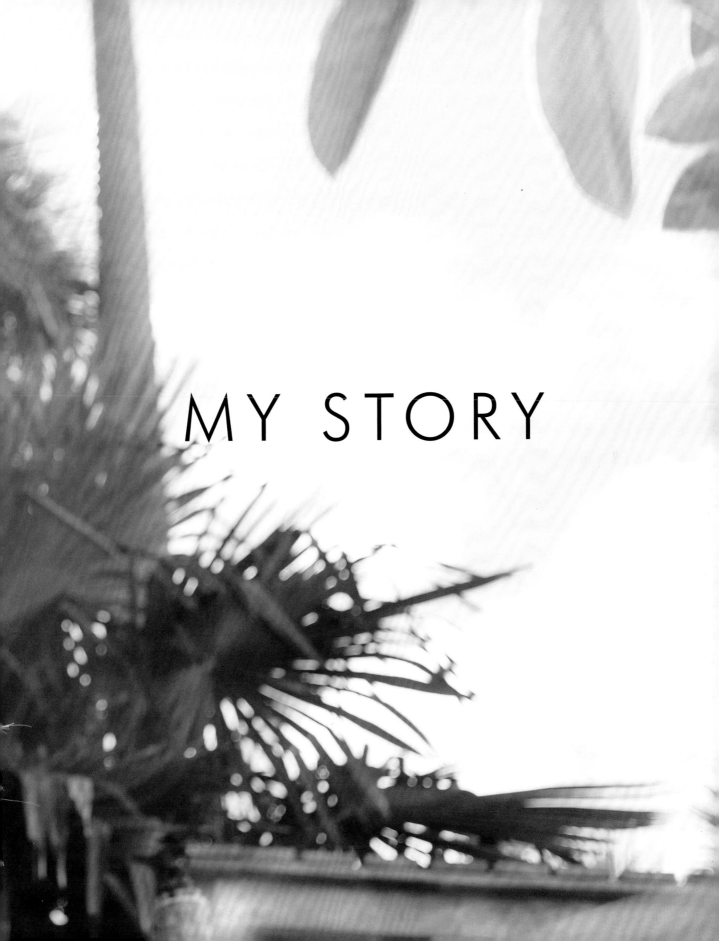

MY STORY

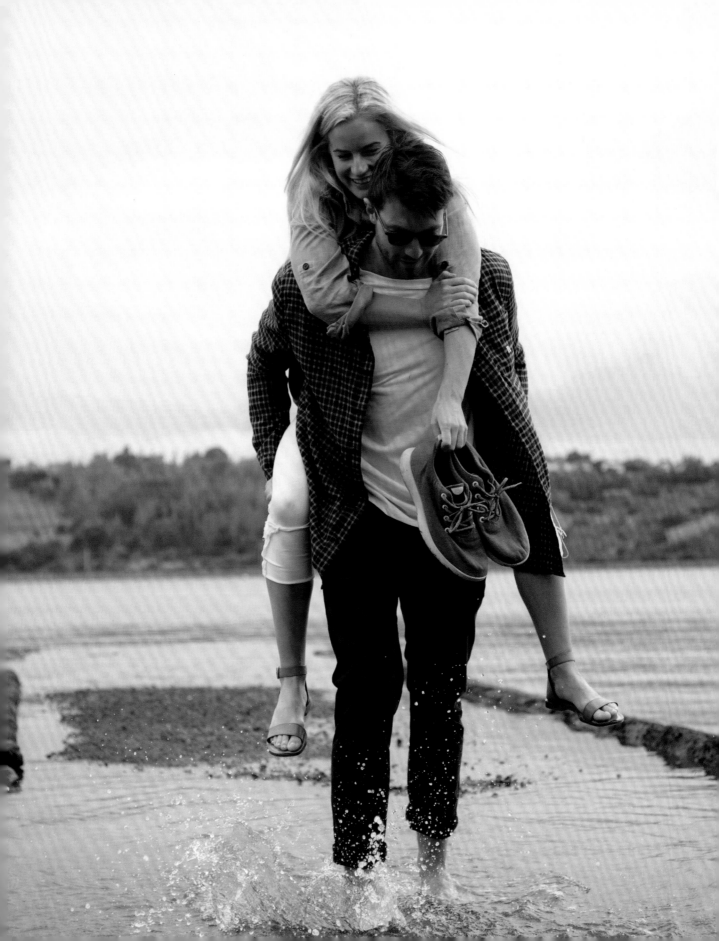

BARE FEET AND MUDDY TRUCKS

I was born in Wahroonga, a suburb of Sydney, Australia, in 1990. I lived there with my parents and my older sister, Chloe, until I was around five years old, when my family decided to move to Waiheke Island in the Hauraki Gulf, about 20 kilometres away from Auckland. My mum is a Kiwi (she was born in Lower Hutt), hence the move back across the ditch. I know what you're thinking: *She's Australian?!* Allow me to explain. Yes, I was born there, but I definitely call myself a Kiwi, since I've lived in New Zealand for 90 per cent of my life and I support the All Blacks (much to my Australian dad's horror).

Growing up on Waiheke Island was a dream childhood. It was incredibly laid-back, and none of the kids at school wore shoes because it was considered uncool. Mum used to force me to wear my shoes to school, but I would hide them in a bush as soon as she had dropped me off. I didn't actually like having bare feet all that much (sensitive soles, you see), but as a child your main fear in life is appearing uncool.

Chloe went to boarding school in Masterton and Mum commuted on the ferry into Auckland each day, so Dad stayed home to look after me for most of my primary-school years. I have such fond memories of that time. I really cherish those years that Dad and I got to spend together. We were best mates. When it rained, there was this road by Surfdale Beach that used to always flood, so as a treat, on our way to go and pick Mum up from the ferry terminal, Dad would drive through the deep puddles at top speed in his Toyota Hilux. Water would splash all over the car and it was *awesome*! I would make him go back and forth a few times until we really had to go and get Mum.

I went to high school in Auckland, so I commuted into the city on the ferry each day, which I loved. The Waiheke commuters all know each other; it's like this little community of pals who catch up twice a day. I made friends with this lovely older lady who taught me how to crochet. (If you're reading this, lovely older lady, I've forgotten how to do it, so could you please get in contact so we can reinstate our lessons?)

After I'd been at high school for a couple of years, I started to notice that my parents didn't seem very happy together any more. They would argue over everything, and I would always hear them fighting after I'd gone to bed. One weekend when Chloe was home from boarding school, we were watching TV together in the living room when Mum came in with a bunch of bags. She gave us a big cuddle and a kiss, and told us that her and Dad were going to split up. She explained that she was going to live somewhere else for a while until they'd had a chance to figure out what was going to happen. I wasn't really old enough to completely understand the situation, so it took me a while to comprehend what was going on.

I think any blow like that to a family takes a long time to recover from. I feel for kids dealing with their parents getting a divorce; it can be a bloody confusing and difficult time. It took me years to fully understand it and come to terms with it. As a kid or young adult you can feel like everything is about you, but as you get older you start to realise that sometimes things just stop working as well as they used to. Now I know that my parents are far better off apart, and I'm so glad that they have each found happiness in their own lives separately—but I do still sometimes wish we could all just sit down and have a meal together. In reality that would probably be more awkward than being forced to sit there while people sing 'Happy Birthday' to you, and there are not many situations more awkward than that.

School wasn't really for me . . . I mean, I loved hanging out with my friends and eating mince-and-cheese pies and Moosies from the tuck shop, but when it came to actual school work I just wasn't into it. By the time I got to Year 13 (my final year of high school), I really couldn't be bothered any more. I found it difficult to focus on subjects that I wasn't passionate about, such as maths and accounting. I loved English and media studies, but unfortunately those were the only subjects I really put a lot of effort into. Once I was in the downward spiral of being behind with my homework and my assignments everything just got worse. I'm pretty sure I had some form of ADHD . . . or maybe I was just a bit lazy. I'm not sure.

Dad, Mum and a very little me. Dad had a pretty impressive mo' on him!

Me in my kindy's production of *Where the Wild Things Are*. Bit cute, right?

24

Anyway, halfway through Year 13, I applied for—and eventually got—a job as a receptionist at a media company in central Auckland. I still remember breaking the news to my parents that I was leaving school. Mum was slightly more understanding, but Dad took a bit longer to come to grips with it, as I had told a little porky and said I already had the credits I needed to go to university (very naughty!). When Dad found out that was a lie, he was a bit disappointed. He eventually came around when he began to understand that I wasn't getting much out of school and wanted to try my luck in the workforce; there was something inside me that knew it was the right path for me. I originally planned to go to university after working for a few years . . . but that never quite happened. My route is definitely not the path for everyone, but I have no regrets.

Working at a media company as a seventeen-year-old was a lot of fun. I made some great friends and it was basically like the fun bit of school where you get to hang with your mates with a bit of work thrown in here and there. Over the next couple of years I moved up the ranks in the sales team, but by the time I turned nineteen I was in a bit of a rut when it came to my personal life. I never had any money, was in a heinous on-and-off relationship with a guy who wasn't very pleasant, and spent my weekends drinking and going to nightclubs until 5 a.m. I ate takeaways for breakfast, lunch and dinner, and the remains mostly found their way to the floor of my car. I'm not kidding—my car was vile. McDonald's and KFC wrappers littered every surface and it smelled like a dog fart.

That was when I hit rock bottom. I woke up one morning flooded with the realisation that I wasn't motivated about anything: I had no goals, no travel plans, no career drive.

That wasn't the person I wanted to be. I decided it was time for a change.

So I booked a one-way ticket to Melbourne.

BECOMING AN ADULT
(OR SOMETHING LIKE THAT)

I realise that moving cities isn't hugely ground-breaking, but it was a pretty big deal for me at the time. I didn't know a soul over in Melbourne, but I was looking forward to starting afresh and becoming more of an adult. A cleaner, tidier adult . . . hopefully. Growing up with a mum who worked incredibly hard and had built a fantastic career for

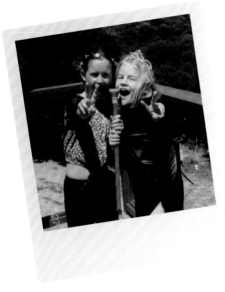

herself, I'd always had this vision of myself doing the same and becoming a real-life 'businesswoman'. I know now that this sounds ridiculous, but I could really picture myself looking all professional in my power suit with my takeaway coffee in one hand and mobile phone in the other. I really wanted to be that woman.

I landed a job at a TV station in Melbourne and worked there for about a year, but I wasn't happy in the role—there was no interaction with other people or time outside of the office, and I found it very claustrophobic. I only had a few friends in Melbourne (and most of them were also my flatmates), and I never felt completely at home. So I did it again. I booked another one-way flight, this time to London.

London was a *whole* different kettle of fish. Anyone who has lived in London with not much money will know that it is a tough city that can chew you up and spit you out when it's done with you. That being said, I had an absolute ball there. I travelled around Europe, sampling all of the bedbug-ridden hostels, gained 10 kilos, landed an amazing job in media at a crime-drama TV channel and ate roast pork at every opportunity. I love the English breed. They are absolutely hilarious and I enjoyed many hours at the pub, laughing with my workmates.

Then in 2013, after four years of living overseas, I felt like I was ready to come home to little ol' New Zealand. It was quite intimidating arriving back on our familiar shores, as things had slightly changed—my friends from school didn't see each other as much, my sister was living in Australia and I was unemployed. It was the same place, but just a little bit different.

For a start, the job hunt was tougher than I thought it would be. I have a mantra that everything will always work out eventually. Sometimes it's slightly naive, and sometimes it takes a while for things to work out (that was definitely the case when I came back to Auckland), but most of the time this philosophy serves me well. After a few months of going to the movies by myself at ten in the morning, going for endless walks, applying for hundreds of jobs and pestering everyone I knew to have lunch with me, I finally got a call from the same media company I had left when I moved to Melbourne. They had heard through the media grapevine that I was back in town, and they needed someone to start straight away . . . and there I was, right back in the possie I had left four years earlier. I had come full circle.

———

I HAVE A MANTRA THAT
EVERYTHING WILL ALWAYS
WORK OUT EVENTUALLY.
SOMETIMES IT'S SLIGHTLY
NAIVE, AND SOMETIMES IT
TAKES A WHILE FOR THINGS
TO WORK OUT . . . BUT MOST
OF THE TIME THIS PHILOSOPHY
SERVES ME WELL.

———

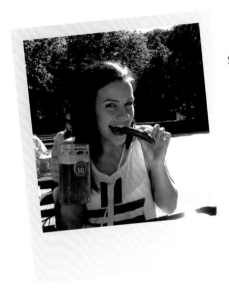

Sampling the local delicacies in Europe . . . It would be rude not to!

HELLO AGAIN, AUCKLAND, MY OLD FRIEND

I worked hard over the next year and a bit, and was really happy. I had a great little flat with two of my best friends, Brooke and Georgie, I was earning enough to enjoy myself, and one of the only things I had to worry about was who was going to mow the lawns. (Georgie, Brooke and I all hated doing the lawns.) I was loving being back home . . . but at the same time I felt like there was a little something missing. So I joined Tinder. Yep, that old chestnut.

Most of my dates were OK. That's it; just OK. I felt as though I was going on a date every week. (That seems to be the way with Tinder: you're either completely committed to getting through every restaurant in the city with a date in tow, or you download the app and never open it once.) But, no matter how many dates I went on, none of them gave me that OMG-I-can't-wait-to-see-him-again feeling. In fact, most of the time I just came home from said dates feeling *meh*. And very full.

One day at work, we found out that there was going to be a Kiwi version of the reality TV-show *The Bachelor*. I had watched the Australian version religiously—I loved it—so I was naturally very excited to hear this news. My manager turned and said to me jokingly, 'Ha, with all the dates you're going on, you should apply!' But when he said it out loud it didn't actually sound that silly. I looked at him, as though to say, 'Should I actually?' and he looked at me, as though to say, 'Maybe you actually should . . .'

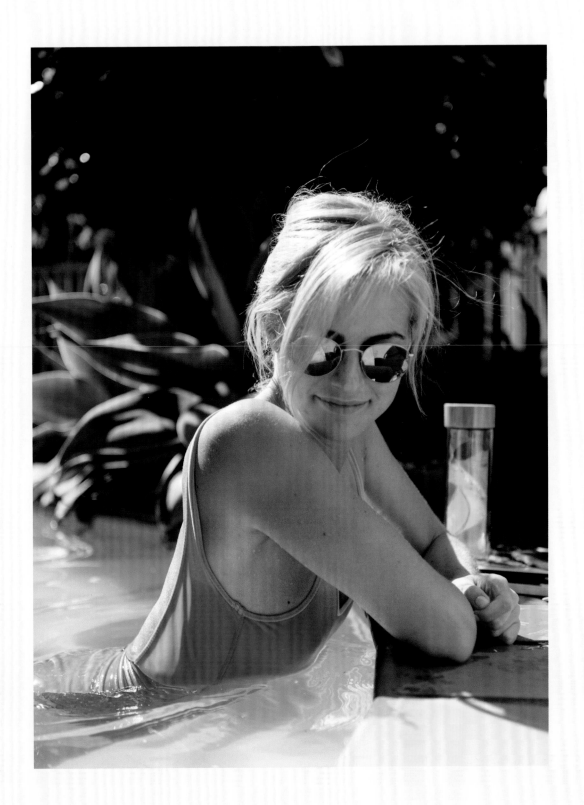

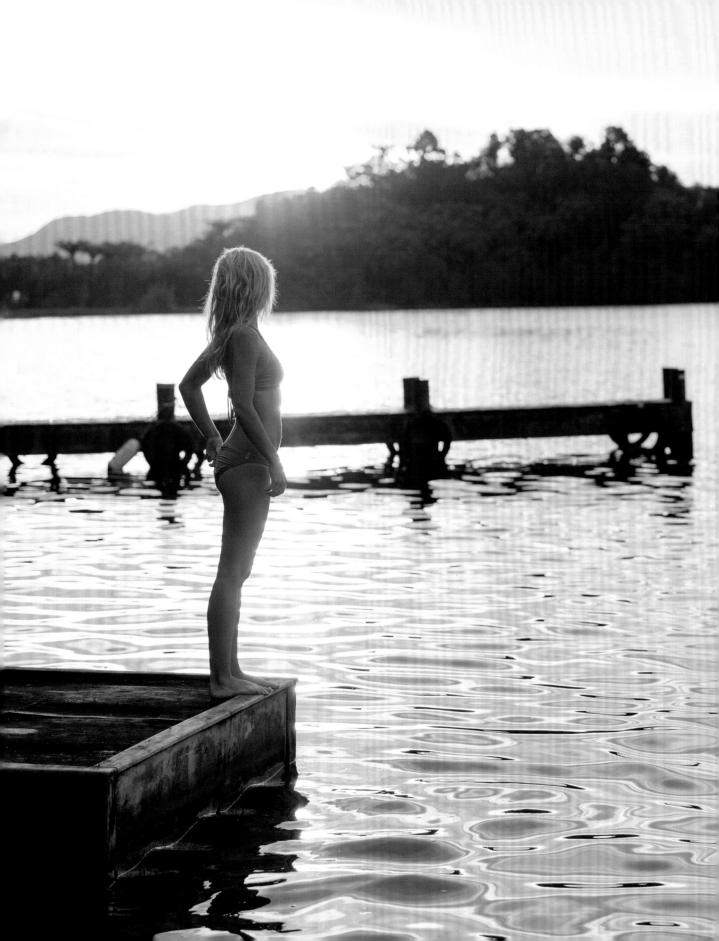

I didn't really have anything to lose, so I decided why not? It might be fun.

Once I got the green light from the big bosses at work (I would need time off if I got on the show), I decided to put in my application, then think more deeply about it if I got a call back.

A few months passed by and I had completely written it off, assuming I hadn't been picked. Then one day I checked my voicemail. Now, I'm one of those really annoying people who pretty much never listens to their messages. If you fail to check more than two voicemail messages, then things are too far gone, in my opinion; by that stage, if you do check them, you're gonna have to go through *all* your messages just to get to the most recent one, and who has time for such nonsense? Well, I had 26 unheard voicemail messages. Things had got ridiculous, even for me. It had reached the point where I needed to just bite the bullet and get rid of them all, so I could return to ignoring my messages like normal.

I made my way through the usual ones from Dad—you know, 'Hi, darling. It's me. Just checking in . . .' There were five of those. Then I hit one that was a voice I didn't recognise; it definitely wasn't Dad.

'Hi, Matilda!' the voice said. It was very upbeat. 'I'm calling from the production team of *The Bachelor*. We loved your application for the show, and it'd be awesome if you could come in for a screen test this week. Give me a call back so we can arrange a time.'

The message had been sitting in my voicemail box for . . . a month. *Oops.*

The next message was from the same person, a week later.

'Hi, Matilda.' The voice was still upbeat, but a little bit less so than the first message. 'Just following up my call from last week. You might have missed it, but we'd still love you to come in for a screen test. Give me a buzz when you have a moment.'

Oh dear.

Then there was a third message, from the week after that. In this one the voice even sounded a little bit annoyed, like I was wasting their very expensive time!

'Hi, Matilda. Just calling one last time, in case you haven't got my other calls. I'll take your silence as you not being interested in being on the show. It would be great if you could let me know either way.'

Crap.

I called back straight away, deeply apologetic.

I was super lucky. They managed to fit me in for a last-minute screen test.

Then, next thing I knew, it was 16 January 2015 and I was getting picked up from my house by a production runner to start my 'journey' on *The Bachelor*.

THE REALITY OF REALITY TV

The whole experience of *The Bachelor* was quite surreal, to say the least. It's hard to explain to anyone who hasn't been through it themselves (which is pretty much everyone), but being in a bubble for two months without contact with anyone outside (which meant no mobile phones or laptops) was quite tough, both mentally and emotionally.

I had about a month to prepare for going on the show. It was one of the hardest secrets I've ever had to keep! I told my family and close friends, as they would have been a bit worried otherwise. It took a while for my family to be totally sold on the concept, mostly because they were concerned that I was opening myself up to criticism from the whole country and they didn't want to see me get hurt. My boss didn't know what to say to my workmates to explain my absence, and ended up telling them that I had gone on holiday to Bali; one of my co-workers in particular thought this was extremely odd, as we had been discussing wanting to go to Bali only a couple of weeks before I suddenly disappeared. The good thing about being on the first season of *The Bachelor NZ*, though, was that, even if people thought my sudden disappearance was a bit odd, no one suspected that I was actually being filmed on top of the Harbour Bridge post-bungy jump.

The two months of filming were an absolute whirlwind. From kissing in front of a bunch of cameras and an entire crew (super awkward) to falling off a horse and breaking my wrist, all the way through to the final day of filming on the Gold Coast when Art said he wanted to make a go of it with me (in slightly more romantic terms than that), it was like a very intense, emotionally difficult fairy tale. Don't get me wrong, there were of course a lot of positives to the whole thing—incredible experiences and strong friendships—but I also want to be honest.

It wasn't easy for me and Art. I knew I liked him as soon as I stepped out of the car on that first night of filming. We had a two-minute conversation to introduce ourselves before I went into the *Bachelor* mansion, and I remember feeling so relieved that he seemed to be my kind of person: funny, warm . . . oh, and extremely handsome. But, as much as I wished that as soon as the cameras stopped rolling we would be hopelessly in love, that simply wasn't the case. For a start, we couldn't be seen together in public until after the finale had aired. So, for two months, we had to sneak around in order to see each other, and even then we only saw each other once or twice a week. We weren't relaxed together at all, as we felt so much pressure from all angles—both from each other, as we wanted to try to make whatever this was work, but also from the media and

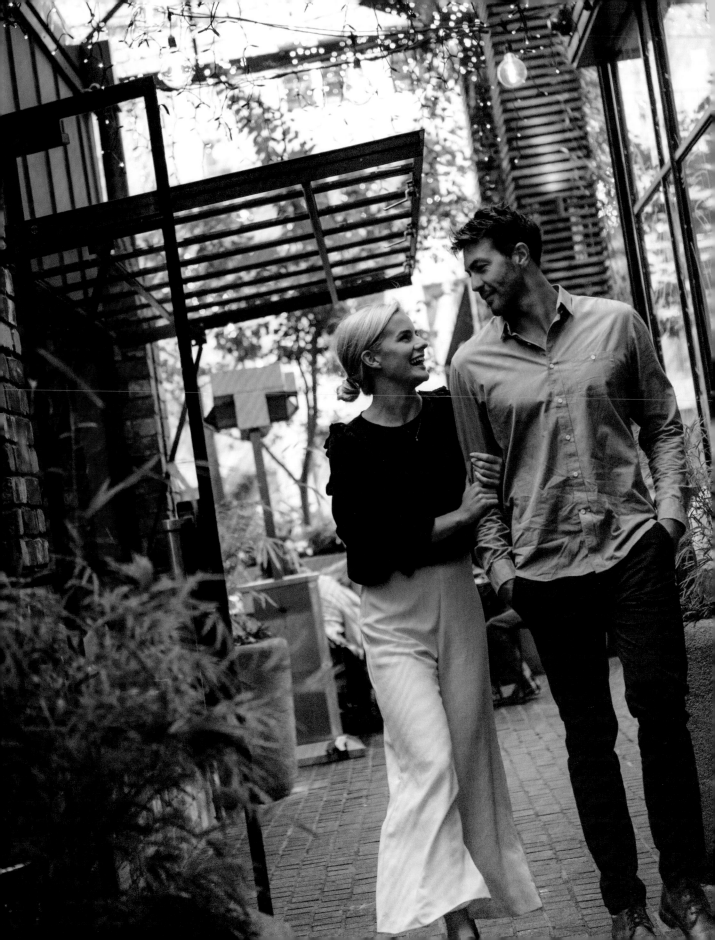

I THINK ART AND I ARE
PRETTY LUCKY TO HAVE A
SOLID FRIENDSHIP AS THE
FOUNDATION OF OUR
RELATIONSHIP. WE HAVE SO
MUCH FUN TOGETHER AND
WE LAUGH EVERY DAY. IN MY
OPINION, IF YOU DON'T HAVE
LAUGHTER, YOU DON'T
HAVE MUCH.

the public. It was a lot to deal with for two people who were just trying to get to know each other.

As soon as we were able to be seen together in public, things became a bit easier. We could start to get to know each other in a far more relaxed way, and we took it slowly—day by day—as the pressure started to ease off. Then, as we grew properly comfortable around each other, our relationship at last blossomed into unconditional love. (Now we are almost *too* comfortable together!)

ONWARDS AND UPWARDS

I think Art and I are pretty lucky to have a solid friendship as the foundation of our relationship. We have so much fun together and we laugh every day. In my opinion, if you don't have laughter, you don't have much.

Life after *The Bachelor* was like another world. Soon everyone was interested in what we were doing and was emotionally invested in our lives, even though we are honestly enormously normal individuals. We were thrown in the deep end in terms of dealing with the media. It was all very new, and we learned from our experiences, good and some not so good, along the way. (*Cough*—Art's controversial costume for a certain Bollywood party—*cough.*)

Our life together now is a lot like that of any other couple around the three-year mark. We are making travel plans. We will eventually get a puppy—it's only a matter of time . . . (That's what I tell myself.) The only difference between us and any other couple, of course, is that you are reading about us.

Also, I've now had enough time in the public eye to have learned how to manage my private and public lives a little better. I'm more careful about what I show on social media, but honestly I'd probably be like that regardless of my circumstances. In an age when everyone shares everything on social media I think it's nice to keep some things private!

Most importantly, I'm excited about what the future holds. Sometimes I get so caught up in my everyday life and work that I forget that I'm still young and I have a whole life ahead of me. I want to travel the world, have a family and go on adventures.

Now I just need to find a way to do everything at once . . .

Challenge accepted.

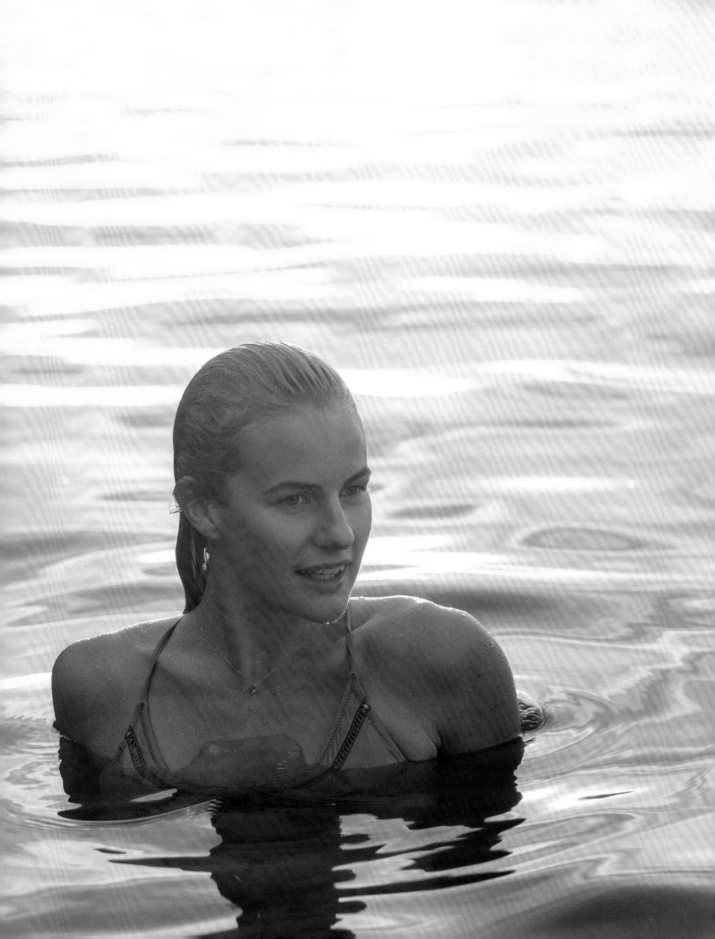

LIVING A
POSITIVE LIFE

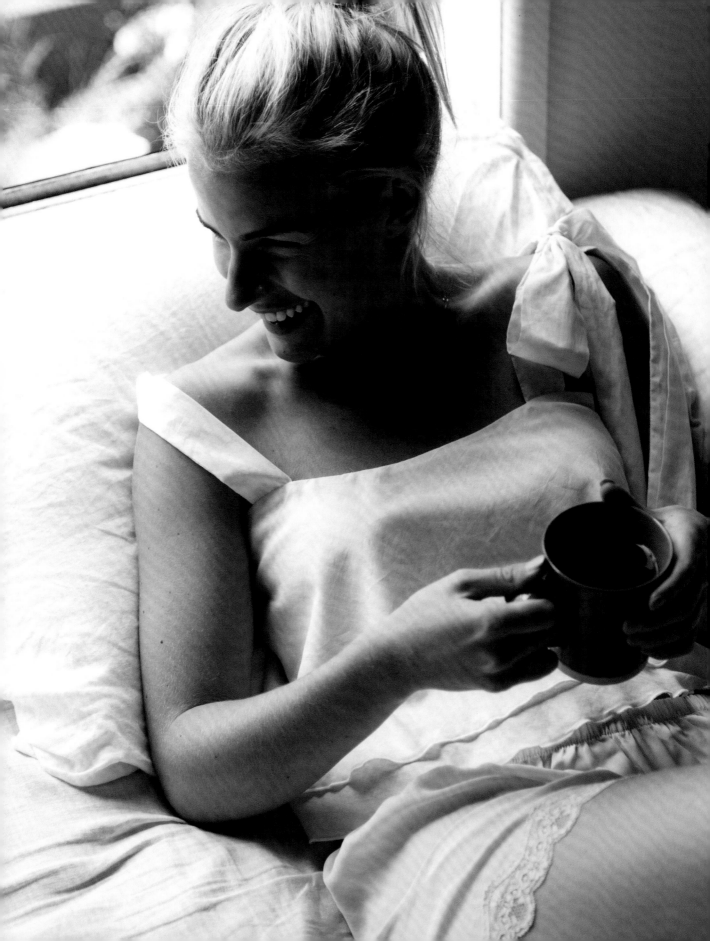

IT WILL ALL BE OK

I like to think of myself as a positive person. As I've mentioned, I've always had the 'it will work out' attitude to life, and I've been lucky that so far it has served me pretty well. I strongly believe that the energy you put out into the world, whether it's positive or negative, determines the type of life you lead, so I work on trying to keeping a positive frame of mind.

Whenever it feels like things are getting the better of me and there's no way out, I tell myself that classic saying, 'Things will be OK in the end, and if it's not OK then it's not the end', and that helps me put things into perspective. I also try to think of the times when I've felt really low and life has been a bit crappy and remind myself that I came out of them unscathed and stronger, and that gives me faith that I'll be able to do it again.

I've found that when you rid yourself of negative thoughts and energy, life seems to improve—more opportunities, more experiences, stronger friendships—all because you're simply concentrating on letting positive energy into your mind, and on looking at the positive aspects of new things rather than the negative. If you focus on finding the positives in whatever life throws at you, you're more likely to go for the new opportunities you are offered.

The annoying thing about keeping your eye on the positive side of life is that it's harder to do some days than others. Life isn't always kind or fair; sometimes it throws you curve balls that can be bloody hard to dodge. It can be difficult to stay positive when it feels like there's nothing good happening in your life (we've all been there at some stage), but the unfortunate thing about negativity is that it's a pretty quick downward spiral: Once you're stuck in that loop, it can be really hard to get out of it and reset, so it's important to recognise when that starts to happen. I say I'm a positive person, and I am—but a positive attitude is also something I try to practise every day. There are a few tricks that I've learned along the way that I find really help with this.

GET A REALITY CHECK

It all comes down to your attitude. Have you ever described someone as having a bad attitude? You know, when someone seems to be deliberately uncooperative, to never want to offer anything constructive, and is negative about everything? I think having a negative attitude about everything is one of the worst traits a person can have, as it affects absolutely *everything*: work, relationships, physical activity and pretty much anything remotely social.

Being positive isn't something I've always been very good at, though. I used to get so frustrated if I wasn't great at something straight away, and I was like that throughout my whole childhood. If I started a sport and wasn't very good (which was the case with pretty much every sport, to be honest; I'm not the most co-ordinated human), then I would give up on it. I'd tell myself that I would *never* be able to do it . . . and then I'd get grumpy about it. When I was at high school, I took up accounting as a subject and, when I didn't quite understand it within the first couple of months, I just gave up on that too. I decided that I couldn't do it, so I just stopped trying, which ultimately resulted in abysmal grades.

The thing is, I had no idea I was so prone to giving up on things I wasn't immediately good at until Art called me out on it one day. I mean, we all know that Art is a fitness machine (it's kind of his thing), so when we started working out together early on in our relationship I didn't like it that much. I always felt like 'the slow one' or 'the weak one', and would inevitably end up in a bad mood that I would take out on the poor boy. He was only trying to help, but he was met with an absolute she-devil in return for his efforts. One day, he bravely decided to mention to me that he was concerned I had a 'bad attitude' when it came to fitness. My first response was stunned disbelief, quickly followed by the thought *HOW DARE HE?!* and I then spent approximately 24 hours thinking he was the rudest of the rude . . . before I realised he might actually be right.

Up until that moment, I had often described other people as having a bad attitude, so having someone—especially someone whose opinion I cared about—say it to me was like a punch in the face. It was a huge reality check that I didn't even know I needed.

Criticism can be really hard to take. Believe me, I know. And, depending on who it comes from, criticism can either be taken with a grain of salt or it can be life-changing. A random person who is mean to you probably has no idea what they are talking about, but if the criticism comes from your family or your friends it's a good idea to at least listen to what they're saying.

CRITICISM CAN EITHER BE
TAKEN WITH A GRAIN OF SALT
OR IT CAN BE LIFE-CHANGING
. . . IF THE CRITICISM COMES
FROM YOUR FAMILY OR YOUR
FRIENDS IT'S A GOOD IDEA
TO AT LEAST LISTEN TO WHAT
THEY'RE SAYING.

What I try to do now is to put myself in the shoes of the person who's offering the criticism; I try to step outside of myself and look at it from their perspective, and ask myself if the criticism is valid. Would I say the same thing to me if I was them? I've found that this is a really good way to figure out if criticism is constructive or not. If you feel it's not constructive, it can sometimes be hard to let it go. Whenever any of us gets a blow to our ego, it takes a little while for the poor thing to mend. I know that 'they're just jealous' can seem like a childish response to criticism, but a lot of the time it's actually quite reasonable. It isn't uncommon for people to feel threatened by someone else's success or happiness, nor is it unreasonable to suggest that some folks feel a certain resentment towards another's motives or ambitions. But my advice is if you're feeling like crap because of someone's unjust criticism just ignore them and keep doing you.

Anyway, it was after the exercise reality-check Art gave me that I eventually realised that I needed to take a look in the mirror. I needed to figure out exactly who I wanted to be.

Did I want to be the person who packs a sad whenever they fail, and just gives up?

Or did I want to be the kind of person who challenges herself and works hard to achieve her goals, even if they seem out of reach?

THE ATTITUDE RESET

Ever since I made my decision about what kind of person I wanted to be (I chose the 'setting and achieving goals' option, by the way—in case that wasn't obvious), I feel like I've grown a lot as a person. It didn't happen overnight, but it did happen.

Here's what I did:

- ♡ I started to make more of an effort to listen to my subconscious.
- ♡ I tried to begin to recognise when I was being unreasonable (I think deep down we all know this, but it's stubbornness that stops us from admitting it!).
- ♡ Instead of responding in a knee-jerk fashion to criticism, I tried to get into the habit of taking a moment to pause and think before reacting.

Slowly but surely, I started to work on turning these moments around. Specifically, I would take a deep breath and try to put the situation into perspective. By doing this,

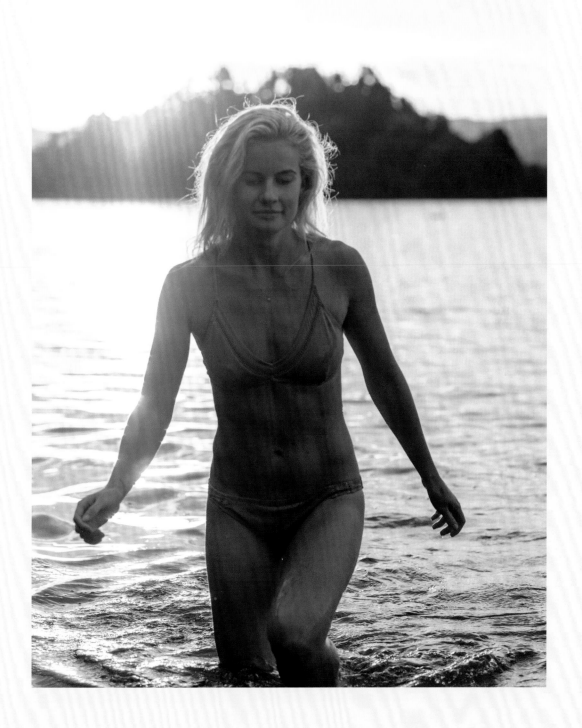

Mood-changers

There are lots of little mood-changers you can use to help you reset your attitude and focus on being more positive about things. My mood-changers include:

♡ taking a deep breath and putting the situation into perspective

♡ faking it until I make it: I put a smile on my face and keep smiling until I actually start feeling happier and more positive (I might look weird, but who cares?)

♡ trying to focus on how far I've come rather than how far I still have to go—it's important to take a moment to remind yourself how much you've improved over time, as it can be easy to forget the progress you've made if you focus on what you haven't done yet

♡ moving! I'll go out for a little stroll and get some fresh air. Even if it's just around the block or up and down the street, it's amazing what a little break and some movement can do

♡ putting on some music and having a dance. I dance all the time, whether it's while making dinner or getting ready in the morning, and I *love* how it makes me feel. It instantly makes me happier and more energised.

Over time, you'll find your own little mood-changers that work for you. Practise them as often as you can and, like anything, you will get better at resetting your attitude. These days I enjoy sports and fitness—and heaps of other things, too—more than ever, all because I have changed my attitude.

I could catch myself (most of the time, anyway) just before I flipped into a bad mood and gave up on everything.

I'm not perfect, but I'm getting better at doing this. The awesome thing is that I feel like I have a far better general attitude as a result. Things don't seem as out of reach as they once did. I'm not as scared as I used to be of trying something new (except perhaps blue cheese; I'm still a bit scared of that). And all of this came from a very simple attitude reset.

It does take time, but the more you work on having a positive attitude, the more natural it will become. If your partner or a friend or family member hasn't confronted you, you may be wondering how to tell if your attitude's a negative one or not. I find that the easiest way to determine if you have a tendency towards being negative is to do the following three things.

1. Step outside of yourself for a moment, and take a look at yourself in the third person.
2. Take the time to analyse how you think from the outside in. Are you always thinking of the negatives first? Do you get upset if things don't immediately go your way?
3. If your answer to either of these questions is 'yes', then make an effort to recognise when you are responding negatively like this, and take some steps to turn your mood around.

TAKE THE RISK

I get scared of taking risks—I think a lot of us do—but I've never really let that stand in the way of me doing something that I know is going to be a good experience. If you feel like you let fear get in the way of doing cool stuff, my suggestion to you is this: when you feel the urge to do something, but fear seems to be holding you back, ignore the fear and go for it!

Nothing compares to the feeling of going ahead and doing something you never thought you could do. When I first moved to London, I was totally terrified. I didn't know a soul over there, and I had gone with hardly any money (I was—and kind of still am, if we're being honest—a terrible saver). But I'll never forget catching the tube to Oxford

Circus when I first arrived, then climbing the steps out of the bustling station and on to Oxford Street, with all its shops and traffic and people. There was so much going on—so many people, jostling and shoving, so many sounds and sights and smells. It was completely different to home. It was overwhelming, but it was also amazing. As I strolled, I gazed around in utter disbelief: I'd actually made it. I'd done it! I was 100 per cent independent in that moment. It was truly liberating.

Of course, there were also times in London when I wished I hadn't taken that risk—I definitely went backwards financially and at times I got really lonely—but when I look back, I wouldn't change it for anything. Throwing myself into a situation where I suddenly had that level of independence taught me a lot, mostly how to 'adult' and be completely self-sufficient. I spent so much time enjoying my own company while exploring the city; I never would have done that if I had stayed in Auckland. It was a bit of an *Eat, Pray, Love* situation: I feel like me, myself and I really bonded during those couple of years. Now we're besties.

Of course, the very meaning of taking a risk is that you don't know what the outcome will be; usually you don't really know if the risk is going to pay off or if it's going to blow up in your face, and that can be scary. But we learn from taking risks—the ones that work as much as the ones that don't—and those lessons can often lead you on to an important new path.

There's a great saying that 'you only learn when you are at risk', and I have personally found this to be spot on. I sometimes wonder how different my life would be—and what kind of a person I would be—if I had never taken some of the risks I have. Once you have started to get into the swing of taking a few risks every now and then, you break free from the average way of living and thinking. You start to gain the momentum and confidence needed to welcome new opportunities into your life. Taking risks builds your self-confidence and self-respect, empowering you to feel stronger and more confident in taking on new endeavours, which—for me, at least—results in a much more positive lifestyle. When you are open to new challenges, you position yourself to gain a whole lot more than you would if you just kept doing the same thing. Plus it's usually much more fun!

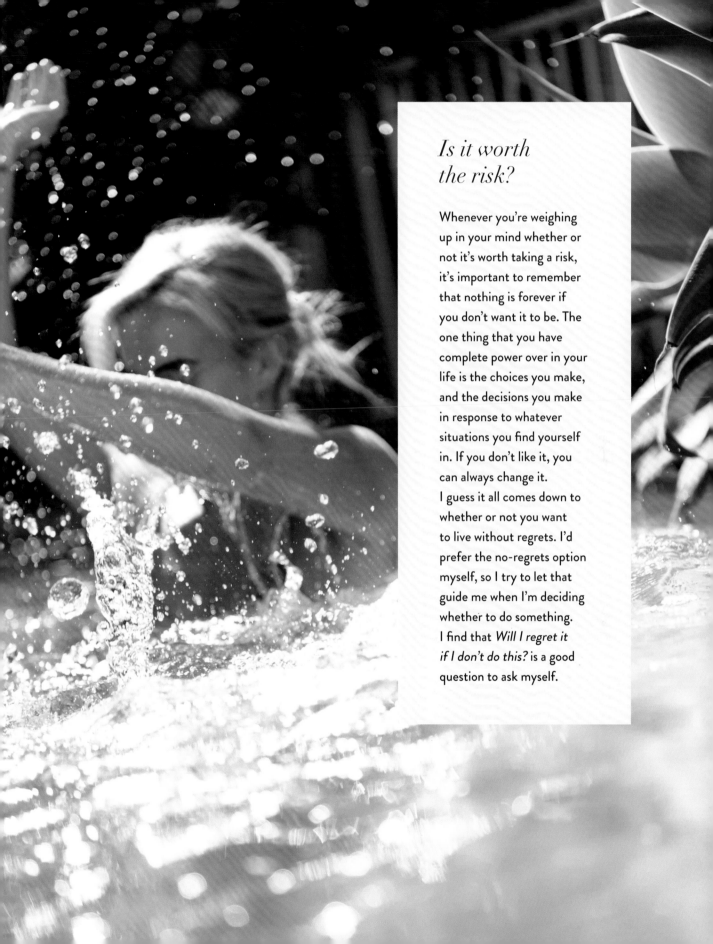

Is it worth the risk?

Whenever you're weighing up in your mind whether or not it's worth taking a risk, it's important to remember that nothing is forever if you don't want it to be. The one thing that you have complete power over in your life is the choices you make, and the decisions you make in response to whatever situations you find yourself in. If you don't like it, you can always change it.
I guess it all comes down to whether or not you want to live without regrets. I'd prefer the no-regrets option myself, so I try to let that guide me when I'm deciding whether to do something. I find that *Will I regret it if I don't do this?* is a good question to ask myself.

LET IT GO . . .

If you're looking to lead a more positive life it's important to let go of grudges. It takes far more effort and emotional energy to harbour anger or negativity towards someone else than it does to forgive them and move on. Have you ever had an argument with someone, or got annoyed at someone for something they've done, and it's all you can think about? I know I have, but ain't nobody got time for that!

I've found that it always helps to look at the true intentions behind the other person's actions. I try to ask myself:

♡ Did their behaviour come from a place of love, or from a place of hate?
♡ Were they trying to make me angry— or were they just trying to help?

Get rid of that grudge

Grudges often arise from things not going how you wish they would. You'll pretend you're fine about it, but you're not really! A big part of getting over grudges is accepting that there are things in life you can't control, and you especially can't control other people. So, instead of focusing on things you can't change (such as other people's behaviour), try to focus on the things you *can* change (your own behaviour). This super-simple action has helped me to develop the ability to brush things off and let things go.

I find that asking myself these questions helps me let things go. I always notice that as soon as I let go of any resentment I'm holding on to it's like a weight has been lifted off my shoulders.

Let's put it into a work context. You've gone for a new role, and bloody Darren, the most annoying guy in the office, gets the job over you. You can either:

a) hate Darren for the rest of your working life, and blame him for something he has no control over (which in turn, will affect your attitude at work), or

b) congratulate him and work harder for when the next role opens up.

Life is far too short to hold on to resentment. I know that letting go of a grudge can be a lot easier said than done, but if you can make baby steps in that direction, then you're on the right track to having a more positive attitude.

———

IT TAKES FAR MORE
EFFORT AND EMOTIONAL
ENERGY TO HARBOUR ANGER
OR NEGATIVITY TOWARDS
SOMEONE ELSE THAN IT
DOES TO FORGIVE THEM
AND MOVE ON.

———

CHILL

Stress is also a major factor that can affect your positivity in a massive way. We've all been there. Stress is always going to be a part of life to varying degrees—you might have an unexpected mechanic's bill or a super-tight deadline at work, or you might be stressed about money being tight or feeling like you never have enough time.

I totally get it, and it sucks.

Stress actually causes a physical response in your body, which can be detrimental to your health if prolonged. Here's where I get all science-y on it, and I bet you're going to think I'm quite smart.

So, your central nervous system (or CNS, for lazy purposes) is in charge of your fight or flight response. Your CNS instantly tells the rest of your body what to do when it encounters a stressful event, herding all resources in your body to combat the cause. (I like to think of it as a little tiny team of people in there directing all the different departments, but that's just me.)

In your brain, the hypothalamus (the part that controls the nervous system, and is also involved in sleep and emotions) gets the ball rolling, telling your adrenal glands to release adrenaline and cortisol. This is a totally natural and vital response that helps us out if we are ever faced with imminent physical danger, like preparing to have a fight (probably a hangover from caveman days). The problem, of course, is that your body can't actually tell the difference between *real* physical-danger type of stress and *perceived* stress—you know, the stress that comes from a deadline at work or ten bills that need to be paid all at once.

As soon as the threat—perceived or real—is gone, your CNS (or team of tiny people) is meant to tell all bodily systems to go back to normal. Everyone has done their job. But, if the CNS fails to return to normal, or if whatever's causing the stress doesn't go away, it starts to take a toll on your body. Symptoms of chronic stress include:

- irritability
- anxiety
- depression
- and sometimes headaches or insomnia.

In other words, not nice. That's why trying to keep stress as low as possible (though of course you will always have some) and developing techniques to deal with it are critical to achieving a more positive lifestyle.

Of course, there can be 'good' stresses and 'bad' stresses in life, and it's important to recognise the difference. For example, a good stress might be something that is challenging but will be rewarding at the end—like running a marathon or throwing yourself into a creative project (like writing a book!) that you know will mean a whole heap of work and a bit of stress thrown in, but will turn out amazingly (hopefully).

Bad stresses, on the other hand, can be really awful things that I wouldn't wish on anyone, like a loved one falling ill, being over your head in debt or going through a break-up that makes you feel like you will never be happy again (spoiler alert: if this is you right now, you will). These bad stresses are the ones that can start to have an effect on your well-being, and it's really important to recognise them early so you can put steps in place to deal with them.

I've listed some of my go-to steps for managing stress over the page. These are things that really help me if ever it all feels like too much, or if I feel as though stress is starting to take its toll on my body. I find that I tend to get stressed or overwhelmed quite easily if I have a lot of work on. I can get so stressed about where to begin that I procrastinate, which just leads to more stress. It's a vicious cycle!

Also, don't forget that chronic stress can be a factor in some other destructive behaviours like overeating or not eating enough, alcohol or drug abuse, or social withdrawal. In a nutshell: try to get that stuff out of your life as quickly as it wrangled its way in there! Hopefully these tips will help you as much as they help me.

My Chillsville playlist

'Let It All Go'—RHODES AND BIRDY
'Girl with the Tattoo'—MIGUEL
'Winter'—MATT CORBY
'Don't Forget About Me'—CLOVES
'Torn'—JAMES TW
'Smoke'—LUKE LEVENSON FEAT. ABBY SMITH
'Ultralight Beam' (Kanye West cover)—EMIR TAHA
'Somebody Else'—THE 1975
'Atlas Hands'—BENJAMIN FRANCES LEFTWICH
'Cherry Wine' (Live)—HOZIER
'Autumn Tree'—MILO GREENE
'Old Pine'—BEN HOWARD
'Ends of the Earth'—LORD HURAN
'Mess Is Mine'—VANCE JOY
'Ritual Union'—LITTLE DRAGON
'Pink + White'—FRANK OCEAN
'In the Morning'—NAO
'Innerbloom'—RÜFÜS
'Free My Mind' (RAC Remix)—KATIE HERZIG
'Just Like Heaven'—THE CURE

MY GO-TO STRESS-LESS STEPS

1. Go for a walk

I know it sounds boring, and you probably think it won't change anything, but I promise that getting outside for a walk does wonders for your mindset. If I ever feel overwhelmed, I'll just chuck on my walking shoes, put on my Chillsville playlist on Spotify and stroll it out. Fresh air clears my mind and helps me to un-jumble my head and figure out a game plan for how I'm going to tackle whatever stress it is that I'm facing. Alone time is important, as it gives you a chance to really think things through without any distractions, and helps you to reboot your brain and unwind.

2. Practise the 'legs up the wall' yoga pose

This is pretty much exactly as it sounds: lie on the floor with your bottom against the wall and your legs straight up it. I'll try to do this for fifteen to twenty minutes if I'm feeling stressed, as it helps my body relax, calms the mind and helps tap into my 'rest and digest' nervous response (as opposed to the fight or flight one). It is also one of the best ways to help drain tension from the legs and feet—and even the hips, if you elevate them on blocks.

3. Get away for the weekend

If the stress in your life is mounting over a period of time and you feel like you just can't get on top of things, get away from it all for a while. Whether it's a weekend with your besties or a Larry Lonesome one, it's amazing what a different setting can do for your soul. There are so many beautiful places around New Zealand that going away for a weekend doesn't have to be a big palaver. Book a cabin somewhere, take a couple of books, and give yourself some time to reset. If money is tight, you could always borrow a tent off a friend or family member and camp for a night or two—there are heaps of cheap and even free Department of Conservation campsites up and down the country. Oh, and don't check your emails or social media! Save any good pictures for the 'gram for when you get home.

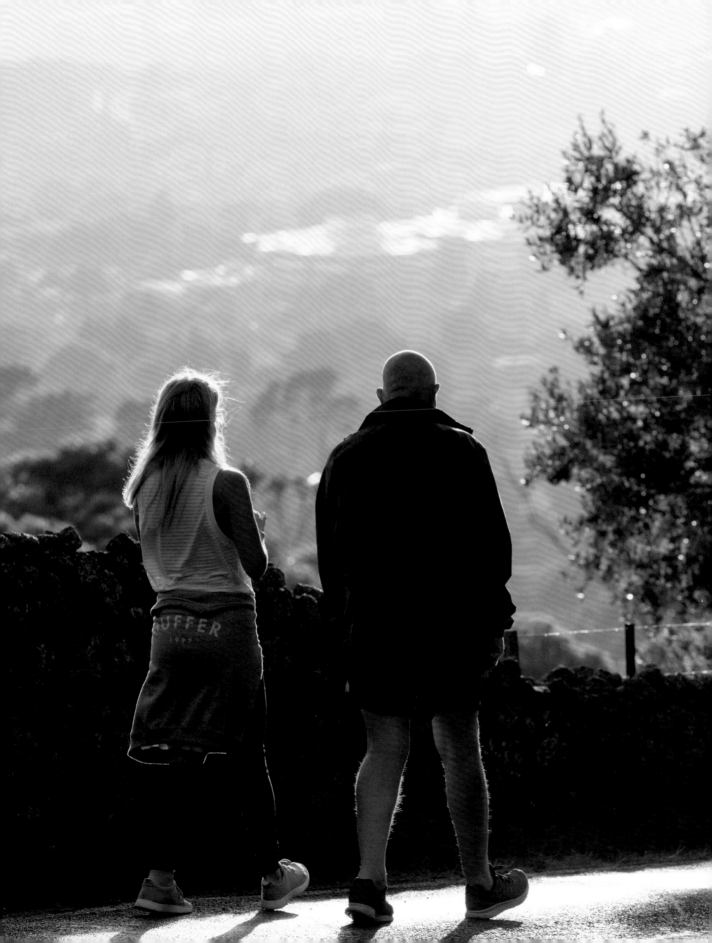

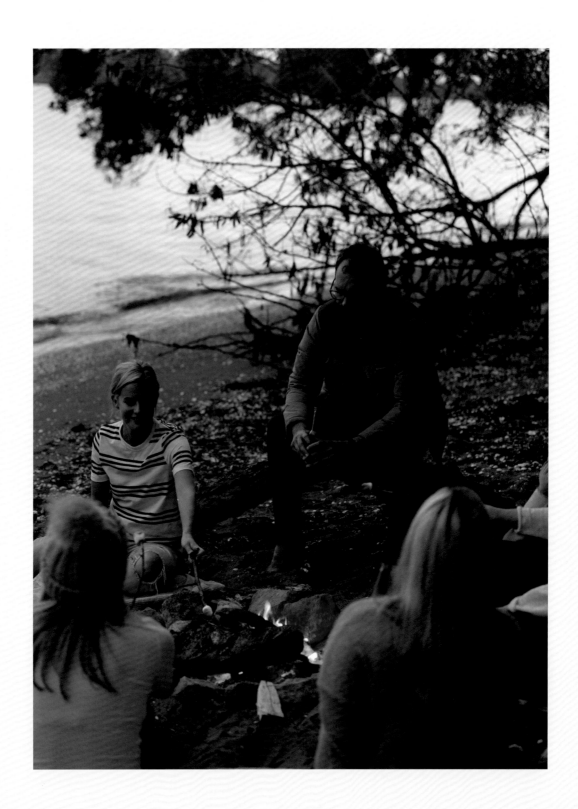

4. Organise a catch-up with your mates

I find that I'm always ten times happier after a good, long catch-up with my friends. We'll get together to chat, laugh *a lot* and solve all our problems over food (and wine). I always come away from these catch-ups feeling refreshed and happy. A catch-up doesn't have to be centred around consuming: you could also organise to go for a walk or run with friends, or play a game of tennis. Sometimes just having someone to listen to you or have a laugh with can be the best medicine.

5. Call your mum

No matter what, mums know best. They have been around a lot longer than you have and chances are they have experienced your exact situation at some stage or another. Any time I'm confused or stressed or overwhelmed, I call my mum and she always knows the exact advice to give for any situation. Mums are just so wise! I hope that if I'm ever a mum I'll be the go-to advice-giver for my kids too. My mum and I have gone through our ups and downs over the years—when I was a teenager, I was convinced she was trying to ruin my life by not letting me ride around in cars with boys or go to parties or whatever, but now I understand it was all because she loves me. We are closer than ever now. As I get older, I find I appreciate my parents for the special people that they are rather than just being my parents. (If you don't have your mum in your life, then go to someone close to you who you look up to—maybe an aunt or uncle, grandparents, or even a friend's parent.)

6. Stop comparing yourself to others

This one is a toughie. I'm pretty certain that every human on this planet compares themselves to someone else at least once every day, whether consciously or subconsciously. Everyone does it; it's kind of a part of life. I think the key is to recognise when you're doing it—and snap the hell out of it! My mum gave me some great advice when I was younger that has stuck with me: 'There will always be someone else who has more than you, and if you compare yourselves to them you will only ever be unhappy. Focus on what you *do* have rather than what you don't.' Don't get me wrong, I still have days when I get frustrated if money is tight, or I get annoyed that I don't have a tummy that's as flat as a pancake, or about the fact that I have no waist (I literally don't: it's just a big square block) . . . but then I think, *Who actually cares?* I would never, ever think that of another person, so I would like to hope that other people aren't thinking that about me. We can be our own harshest judges. And, at the end of the day, I'd way rather take health and happiness over anything else. Sometimes I just have to remind myself of that.

7. Do something nice for yourself

Sometimes it helps to think of what you would suggest or do to help a friend or family member who's going through a stressful time, then apply that to yourself. It could even be something really simple like making yourself a cup of tea and drinking it in bed with a magazine, or binge-watching a season of your guilty-pleasure show (like *Geordie Shore*— that's not just me, right?). You could even take the morning and treat yourself to a mani-pedi or a massage. I mean, how can you beat a massage? They are the bee's knees.

8. Write it down, or talk to a good friend about it

Sometimes just getting something off your chest helps to put it all in perspective. Your own mind tends to make a bigger deal out of things than it needs to, so getting advice from a friend can help you to realise that your stress is not too big to manage. Making lists when you feel overwhelmed can also be helpful for some people. If you've got a big job you're working on, separate it into smaller tasks, then cross them off as you go—this helps me when I can't figure out where to start, which is often!

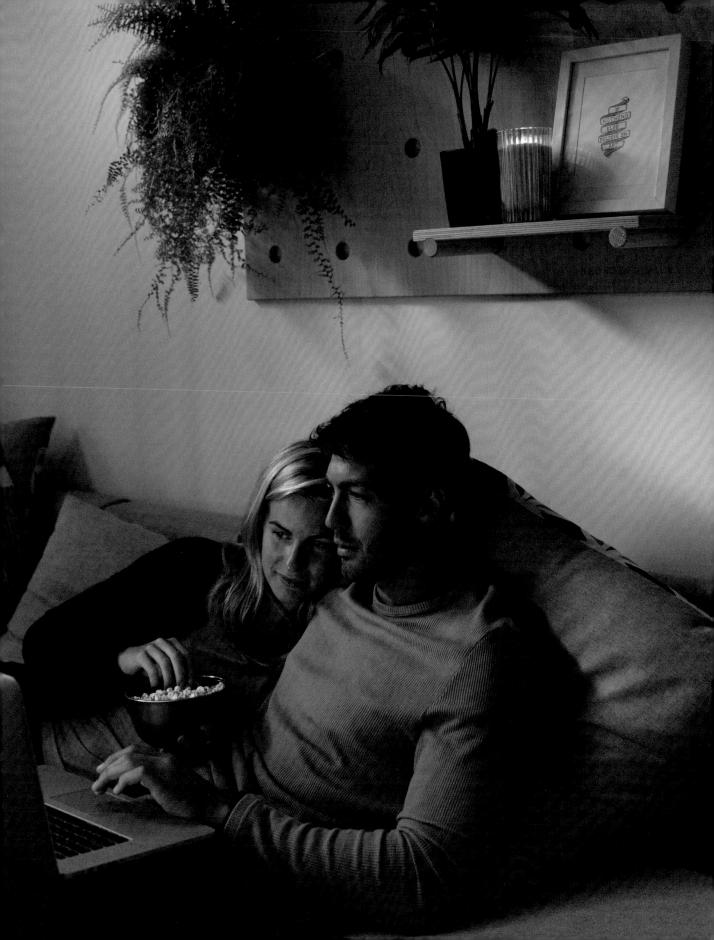

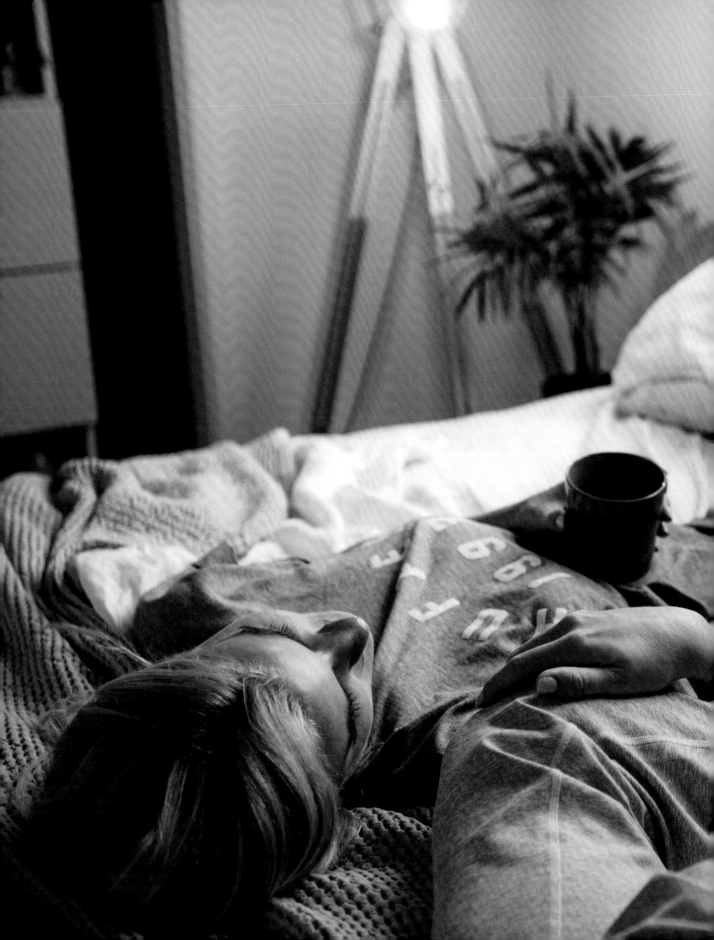

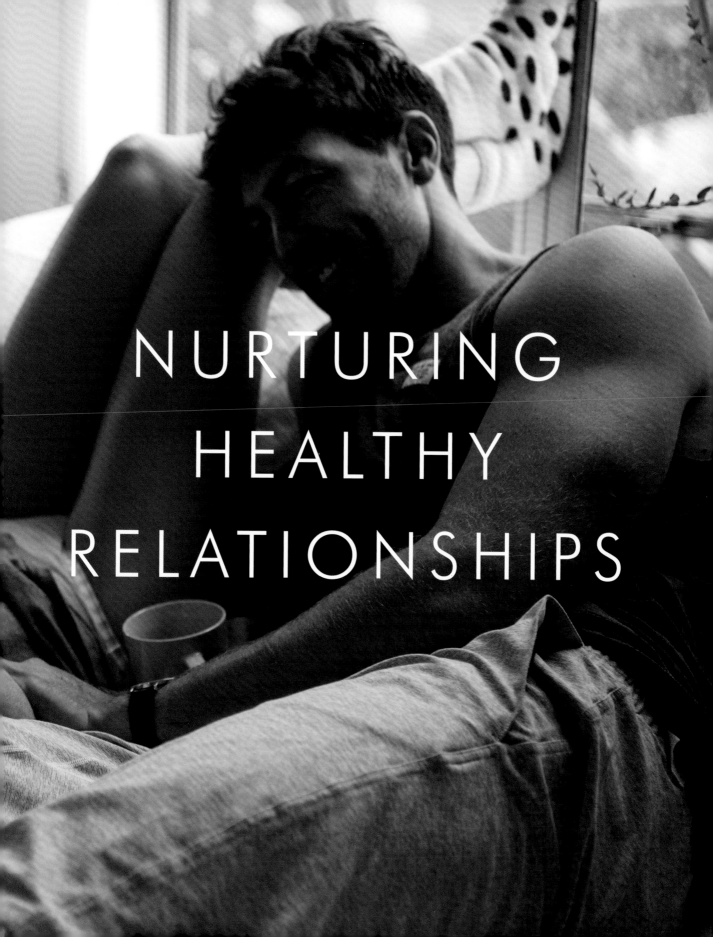

NURTURING
HEALTHY
RELATIONSHIPS

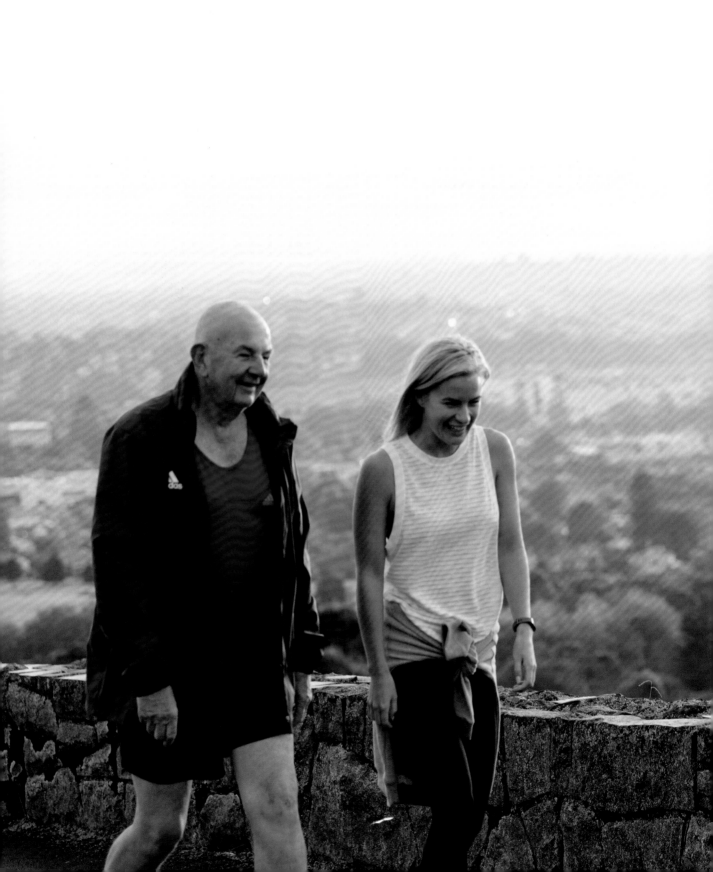

Relationships are a beautiful part of living. They can be hard work, even draining at times, but the joy of other people's company is something we as humans can't live without. Relationships come in all shapes and sizes: there's your family and friends, your partner, your co-workers, even the barista at your local cafe, and of course your relationship with yourself. You have a relationship with all of these people, just to varying depths.

Having positive relationships, and nurturing the relationships that are important to you, is a huge part of leading a beautiful life. When times get tough, your relationships can be a huge source of comfort, happiness and joy. And, when times are good, your relationships are heaps of fun—and being able to share good times only multiplies the goodness!

FAMILY

———————

Let's start with one of the most important relationships: your family. There's an old saying that you can choose your friends, but you can't choose your family. It's thrown around quite a lot—most of you will have heard it at some stage or another—and it is one of those common truths. Whether you get along with your family or not, they are still your family; there's not much you can do about it.

I have a small family and I've always been very close to them. It's just my parents, my older sister, Chloe, and me. My sister is one of the kindest souls I have ever encountered, and she will go out of her way to help anyone in need. She's living overseas at the moment and it's been so long (too long, actually) since we have lived in the same city. We are very close and have always been one another's confidant. She has exactly the same silly sense of humour as I do, so we laugh a lot . . . and I do mean a *lot*.

As I've mentioned, I spent a lot of time with Dad when I was younger and we lived on

Parents: annoying because they love you

One of the cool things about growing up is that you start to see your parents as people in their own right—people who have lives outside of you (I know, unbelievable but true!), who have their own stresses, problems and challenges. You start to understand their strengths and flaws, and appreciate the different qualities they bring to your life.

Your parents are only human, too, after all, and they're usually just trying to do their best. My parents always used to joke that my sister and I didn't come with a manual. I wish I had understood this better when I was a teenager, as it's helped me to see where my parents are coming from and to make our relationship so much better.

If ever I feel frustrated with my parents, I try to put myself in their shoes, and ask myself, *Would I feel the same if I was them?* I also try to remember that they only have my best interests at heart and they are just trying to protect me. It's good to keep that in mind!

Waiheke, and Mum was commuting to Auckland for work. Dad and I would just hang out, go to the beach, drink hot chocolates and eat ice cream. I believe those years shaped our relationship. I see him as a friend, someone I can laugh with, and I know I can always look to him to cheer me up with a good dad joke (usually one that I've already heard a couple of times before). He's a big kid at heart and doesn't take life too seriously. I love that about him.

After my parents divorced, I moved in with my Mum in Auckland and it wasn't long until I became a truly horrific teenager. It's a bit of a cliché, actually. I thought I knew everything and I was convinced that Mum was out to ruin my life just because she didn't want me driving around in cars with boys who didn't have their full licence (which I now know is fair enough!). Our relationship became a bit strained over those years, and we fought a wee bit. When I look back on that time now, I feel so terrible for adding stress that she definitely didn't need to her life.

It can be hard to understand when you're a teenager, but all your parents want is for you to be safe, because they love you more than life itself. Even through those years of me being a difficult teenager (sorry, Mum), my mum was always there for me when I needed her. If I was ever sad or frustrated or confused about something, she would make time for me and help me through it. I've never met anyone as wise as my mum, and I wish I could have appreciated that more when I was a teenager! As I got older (and more mature), our relationship improved and we started to

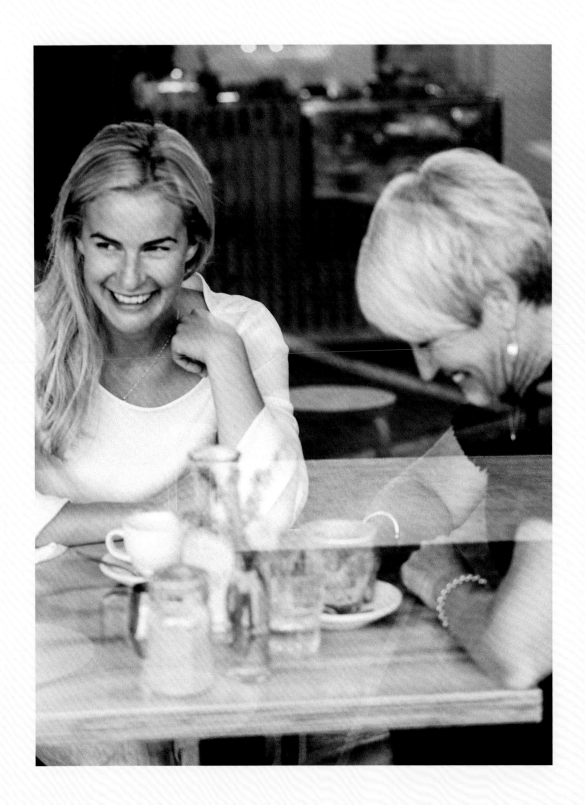

understand each other better. Now, I'm happy to say that we are closer than ever. If I grow up to be half as good a mum as she is, I'll be happy.

Every family is different, but one of the things I love the most about my family is that they will always be honest with me. They are usually the first ones to give me a reality check (see the previous chapter for more on those), but they are also usually the first ones to stand up for me and protect me if anyone's being unkind or unfair. I guess they can sometimes be *brutally* honest, because they know that I love them no matter what— even when they are telling me something they know I probably don't want to hear!

The most important thing to remember is this: cherish your family, because life is short, and you only have one family.

FRIENDS

Friendships are a huge part of your life. I have lots of different friends who I have met through all areas of my life—I've got my school friends, who I love and adore and who know me so well after almost fifteen years, and then I've got friends who I met later in life through work, mutual friends or the gym, and each of whom I treasure individually for different reasons. When I was a teenager, I went to boarding school in Auckland for a couple of years (after I got sick of commuting from Waiheke) and I loved getting to know people who I probably wouldn't have spent much time with otherwise, as we were all in different friend groups at school itself. Then, when I left school it was such a cool feeling to suddenly have a whole bunch of new friendships opening up in front of me; it can be easy to get so caught up in your group of friends at school that you don't really meet anyone new, so it's awesome when the world becomes that little bit bigger through new friends.

The friends you choose to surround yourself with have a profound effect on your happiness, so it's vital that you choose them wisely. Among other things, friendships help you keep your sanity. I have a chat group with some of my friends, and whenever I'm upset, frustrated or just want to share a cute picture of a baby pig, they are there to talk about it and will always make time for me.

Although mostly awesome, friendships can also be tough at times. People go on different journeys in life, or they grow apart, or sometimes you realise that a certain

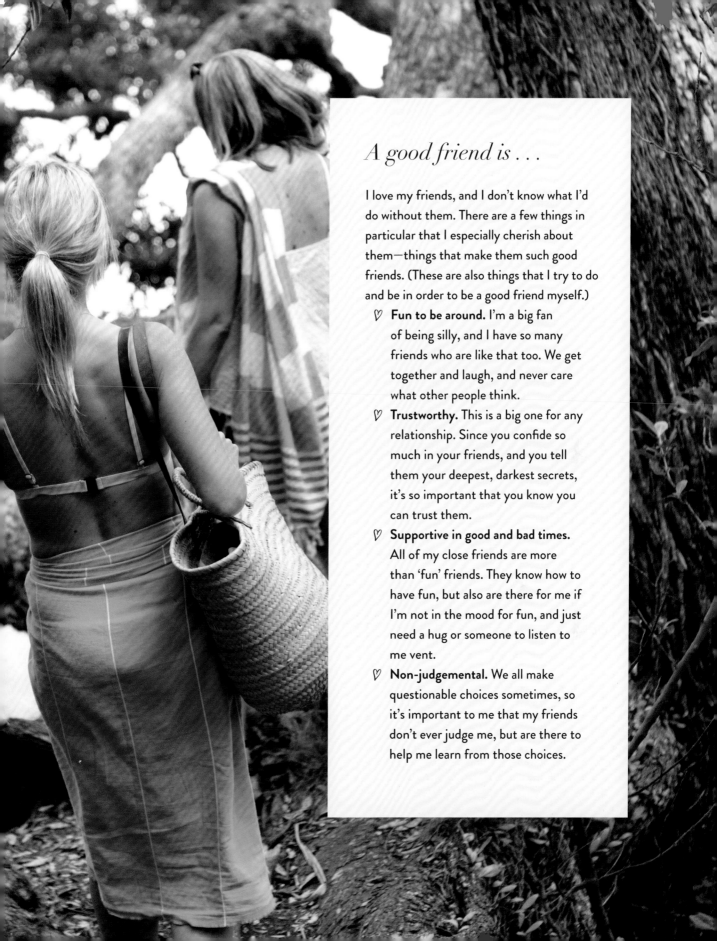

A good friend is . . .

I love my friends, and I don't know what I'd do without them. There are a few things in particular that I especially cherish about them—things that make them such good friends. (These are also things that I try to do and be in order to be a good friend myself.)

♡ **Fun to be around.** I'm a big fan of being silly, and I have so many friends who are like that too. We get together and laugh, and never care what other people think.

♡ **Trustworthy.** This is a big one for any relationship. Since you confide so much in your friends, and you tell them your deepest, darkest secrets, it's so important that you know you can trust them.

♡ **Supportive in good and bad times.** All of my close friends are more than 'fun' friends. They know how to have fun, but also are there for me if I'm not in the mood for fun, and just need a hug or someone to listen to me vent.

♡ **Non-judgemental.** We all make questionable choices sometimes, so it's important to me that my friends don't ever judge me, but are there to help me learn from those choices.

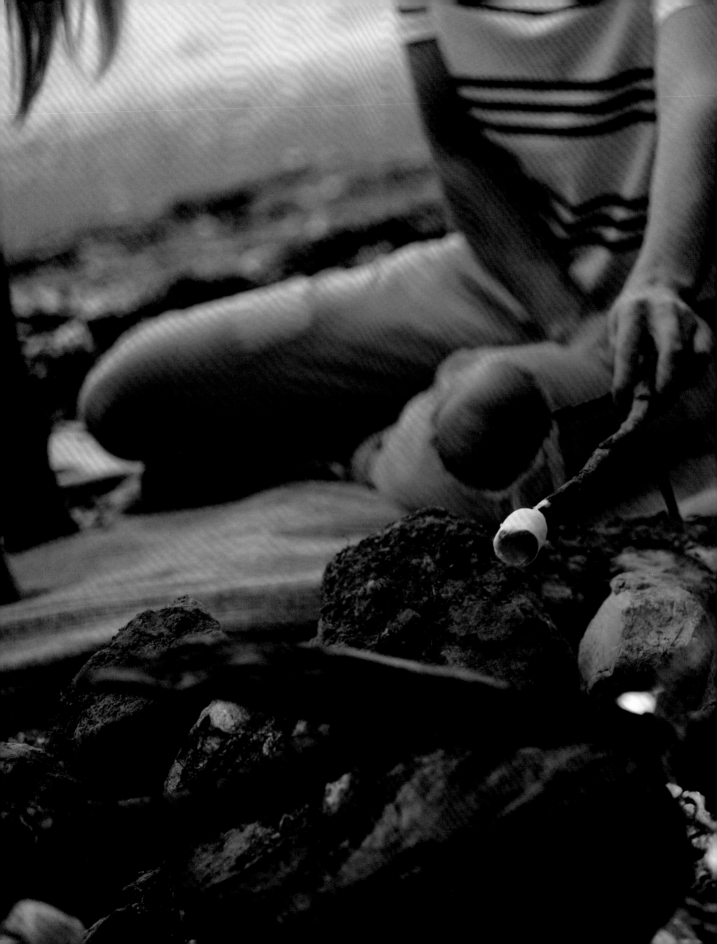

Breaking up with a friend

One thing I've learned in my (admittedly quite short so far) lifetime is that your happiness is heavily affected by the people around you. Your happiness should always be your number-one priority! If you feel like you have a friend who doesn't empower you, or lift you up if you're feeling down, or make you laugh, then maybe it's time to have a think about whether you want that person in your life.

'Breaking up' with a friend is arguably harder than breaking up with a boyfriend or girlfriend, but it is an absolute investment in your long-term happiness and overall well-being. Your self-esteem is precious—it affects every area of your life—so, if there's someone near to you who's compromising that, they have no place in your life. Simple as that!

Some signs that a friendship might not really be so friendly any more:

♡ When you have something on your mind that you want to talk about, your friend seems uninterested and doesn't really listen. People can get caught up in their own lives sometimes, but if this happens all the time then you need to ask yourself if this person really cares about you or is it a friendship for selfish reasons?

♡ The negative interactions outweigh the positive ones. If you find yourself constantly feeling uncomfortable around that person or feeling anxious because of them, then that's a sign that you aren't compatible with them any more (or never were).

♡ There is jealousy and competition. A little bit of healthy, fun competition never hurt anyone, but if your friend is constantly trying to compete with you and one-up you, that may be a sign it's time to call it quits. Your friends should be encouraging you to do well and reach your goals, not be trying to be better than you all the time.

Even if you feel as though a friendship might have run its course, that doesn't mean things have to get nasty. Often it's as simple as just letting a friendship wane on its own—instead of focusing your time on that friend, turn your attention to the ones who nurture and support you and make you feel good about yourself. In a lot of situations, both of you probably realise the friendship isn't working but don't know what to do about it. And who knows? Sometimes you might part ways with that friend for a little while, only to come back to each other later in life as you each grow and get to know yourselves better. People change, and sometimes we all just need a little bit of time.

person doesn't add any love or positivity to your life. That can be a really tough thing to deal with. You invest so much of your emotional well-being in your friendships, but it needs to be returned; it needs to be a two-way street, where you give love and kindness but also receive it.

LOVERS

The exact same thing goes for romantic relationships as for friendships. Art is my first really serious relationship and I can honestly say I'm pretty bloody happy with life these days. I had a few boyfriends in high school, but I found that it was hard to distinguish between genuine attraction and someone who I just thought was 'cool' at that age. I had my fair share of not-so-amazing relationships in my early twenties, but I took lessons away from each one; average relationships can help you recognise and appreciate the amazing ones. I think there's a little corner of your heart that is reserved for that special someone. You don't even know it's there until you've found the right person, then all of a sudden your heart seems bigger than it was before. (Yes, I am a bit of a romantic. Don't judge me. I love a good love story!)

That said, I believe that life is too short to settle for someone who doesn't improve your life in some way. When you're with your partner, you should feel empowered, confident and as though you are enough exactly as you are. So often I see people— women especially—who are constantly trying to be 'enough' for their partner: athletic enough, beautiful enough, whatever-it-is enough. That's not love. You should never have to change who you are to be with someone—and, if you feel like you do, then you need to move on. You're much better to hold out until you find someone who loves you just the way you are. I sometimes wonder if the reason some people don't meet that special person is because they are wasting their time settling for someone who isn't quite right.

If you are single, enjoy flying solo! Being single doesn't have to be the horrible thing it's sometimes made out to be. Hanging out with yourself and doing all the things that make *you* feel good is a way better option than settling for someone who treats you like crap and makes you feel terrible about yourself. You can do whatever you want, whenever you want, without checking in with someone else. That's pretty awesome— like, you could just move to another city tomorrow if you felt like it (hypothetically,

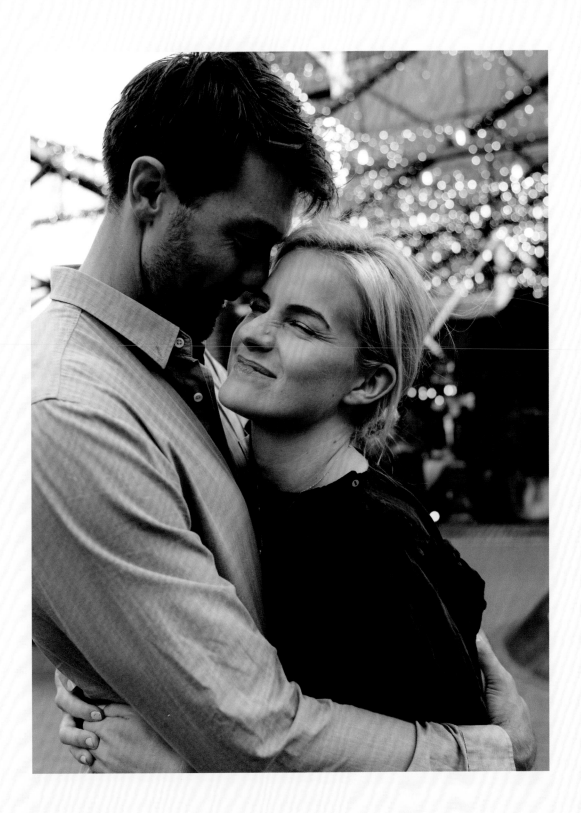

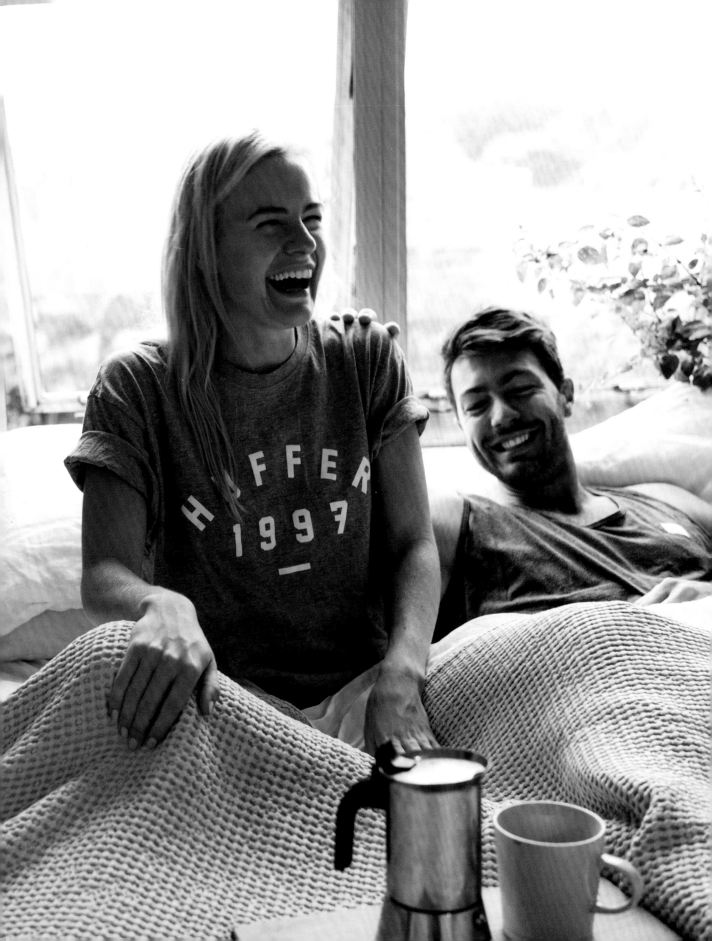

as it would be quite a lot to organise in a day) without having to work in with someone else's schedule.

Even though I'm a bit of a romantic wee soul, I have never believed that you need a significant other in order to be happy. I was lucky that my parents taught me from a young age the importance of keeping your independence, and of carving your own path. I've carried that lesson throughout my life. As a woman especially, your happiness should never be centred around a partner. In my mind, a romantic relationship should be added value to an already beautiful life. One of the qualities that I admire most in other people is the ability to enjoy their own company. It's super cool when someone doesn't need fulfilment from others, but gets it from themselves.

Signs of a good romantic relationship

♡ **You are good friends.** Romance is one thing, but sometimes you just want to call up your lover and tell them a funny story without talking about when you want to get married and have kids. It's important to enjoy each other's company and that your relationship is full of laughter and fun.

♡ **Your communication is on point.** This one sometimes doesn't happen straight away, but it's important that it's there. If you feel like you can talk to your partner about things that sometimes aren't easy to talk about, then you're on to a good thing.

♡ **You have your independence.** Relationships are fun, and when you're in a good one you want to spend all of your time with the other person, but it's important to have your own interests too. Keeping your independence is important so you don't lose who you are just because you are in a relationship.

♡ **Your relationship is your safe place.** It should be your home, and you should feel safe and happy when you are with your significant other.

♡ **You can both say you're sorry.** Everyone makes mistakes, and when you spend so much time with someone you're bound to accidentally hurt their feelings sometimes, so it's important that you are both comfortable with yourselves and can admit when you're wrong.

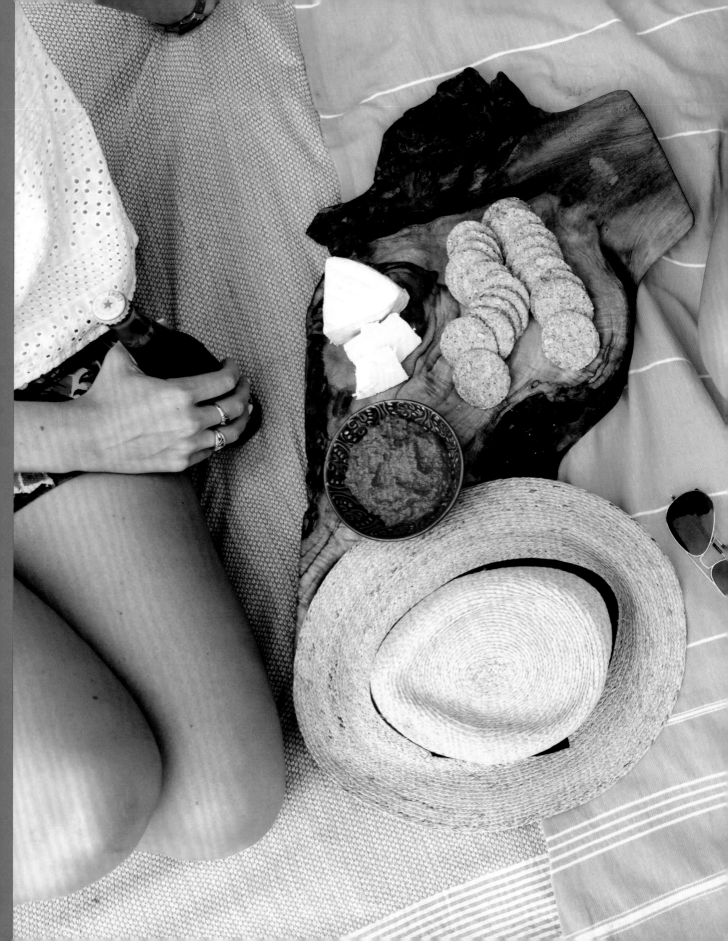

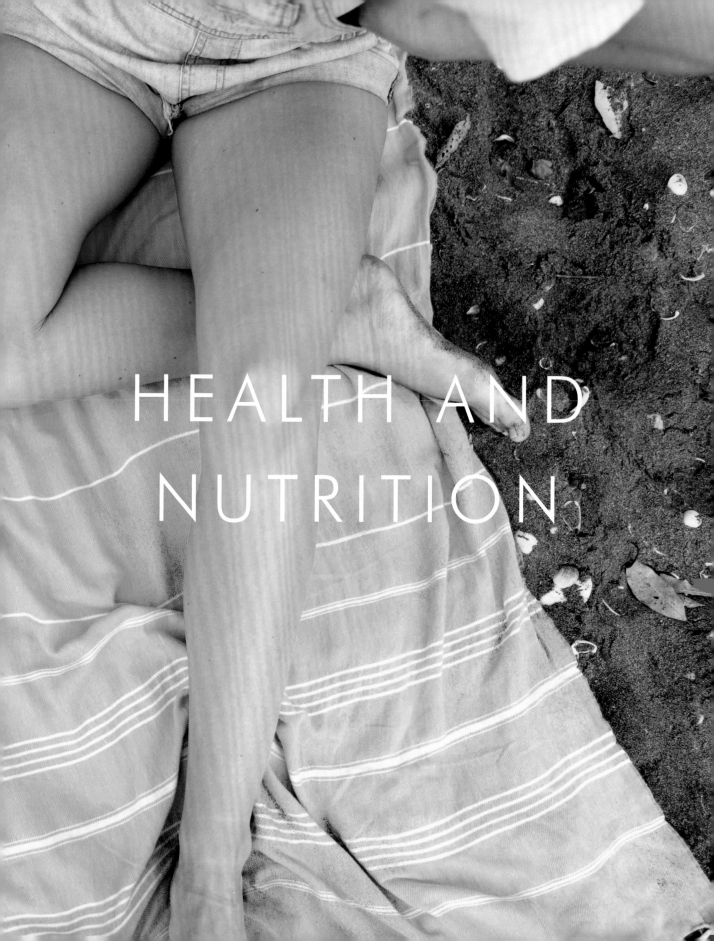

HEALTH AND
NUTRITION

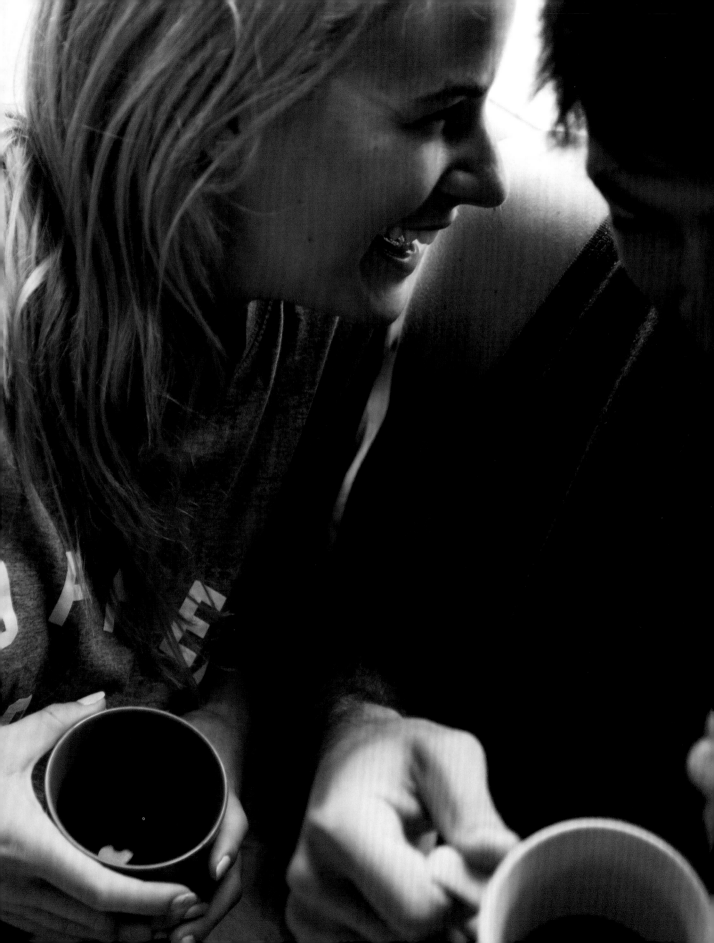

Food. It's everywhere, it's delicious and without it we would die. I love food. Since food is such a huge part of our lives, I think it's extremely important that we enjoy it for the beautiful thing that it is.

WHAT IS THIS 'HEALTHY' YOU SPEAK OF?

I've been through a lot of ups and downs with health and nutrition over the years. Growing up, I was an extremely fussy eater. I had this weird thing about food textures, so I wouldn't eat any fruit or vegetables, which frustrated my parents endlessly (as you can imagine). I remember Dad tried to get me to eat one banana a day, but I caused such a scene about it that he changed it to just one tiny *piece* of banana—and even that was like child abuse! I pretty much lived on spaghetti bolognese and fish fingers (not at the same time of course—that would just be weird). Our family doctor on Waiheke Island used to tell my parents I would get rickets if I didn't eat more fruit and vege. I still eat a lot of spaghetti bolognese now, but not quite as many fish fingers. Oh, and I don't have rickets.

Throughout my high-school years, I ate whatever I liked. I still stayed away from fruit and vegetables, because I was more into KFC and McDonald's. I was naturally slim, so I assumed that I was healthy enough. (Bless, I had no idea.) I moved into my first flat with some friends when I was eighteen, and I don't think we cooked a meal once. It's not much of a surprise that I hardly ever had any energy and found it hard to concentrate.

I continued to live my life that way until I moved to London for the classic two-year stint. While I was there, I travelled throughout Europe and ate all of the pizzas and gyros (can I get a 'hell yeah!' for gyros?) and, in the process, put on a fair bit of chunk. 'You're looking very healthy around the face area,' I remember my mum telling me when I was Skyping her one day. (That was her lovely way of saying I was fat.)

That was the moment I decided to get my act together and start making healthier choices . . . but the problem, I know now with the benefit of hindsight, was that I had no bloody clue about what 'healthy' even was. My idea of a healthy dinner back then was a bowl of iceberg lettuce drowned in sugary dressing. I know, ridiculous.

I began to do some research, and got more and more interested in fitness and nutrition—but then I started taking it way too far. This is such an easy trap to fall into, and it happens to the best of us. Here's what happened.

THE NOT-SO-HEALTHY
SIDE OF 'HEALTHY'

I downloaded an app which was supposed to help you 'lose weight the healthy way'. As well as being a fitness and exercise tracker, it was also a calorie counter. I started documenting *everything* I ate. It reached the point where I would freak out if I went over my measly 1200-calorie daily allocation. This was not good; in fact, it was dangerously low. According to most nutrition guidelines, a woman of my age at the time requires anywhere between 1800 and 2000 calories a day—and that's if she doesn't do any exercise. If you exercise, you (obviously) need to eat more. Apps don't know anything. I don't believe in counting calories any more; if you eat healthy meals most of the time, you will be just fine.

I became so addicted to losing weight that I would avoid social occasions like going out for dinner in case I would have to eat something 'unhealthy'. I know this sounds extreme—and it is—but things snowballed pretty quickly, and I didn't realise how bad things had got. I thought I was doing a good thing by being what I thought was 'healthy'.

On top of this, I also had a trainer who I would see twice a week, and I would only ever eat carbs after I worked out (I was actually encouraged to do this by my trainer—ridiculous). If you do the math, that means I ate carbs only a few times a week.

I did get in great shape—the best shape I've probably ever been in in my life—but

I wasn't happy. I wasn't happy at all. All I ever thought about was food, and if I had one drop of sugar I would binge on it as if I would never eat again. I was also very lonely: as well as being a long way from my family, all my friends lived on the other side of London.

When I look back at that period of my life now, I believe I was depressed. I thought I was the epitome of health, but I now realise that I couldn't have been further from it.

Fast-forward six months or so, and I started eating normally again and it all came back. The weight, I mean. The thing about 'dieting' and restricting your calories like that is it is not sustainable. You can't keep restricting your calories for the rest of your life, because your body is constantly fighting it, so it is only a matter of time before you give in. As soon as I started eating normally again, my body, fearing it would find itself starved of nutrients once more, held on to everything and stored it all as fat. It had learned from last time round, and was getting ready for the starvation!

That's what you're doing to your poor body when you restrict it so heavily. It needs a lot of nutrients to function at the best level it can, and it can only get those nutrients from the food you eat.

Clues things might have got out of hand . . .

♡ **You're secretive about the extent of your dieting.** If you can't be open and honest with your friends and family about what you are *truly* eating because you are afraid of what they might say, then that's a sign you are probably taking it too far.

♡ **You spend most of your time thinking about food.** Don't get me wrong, I think about what I'm about to eat all the time. I *love* food! But if you find it hard to think about anything else, and you're fretting about what you are or aren't eating and whether or not it's 'healthy' enough, then that's not healthy.

♡ **You don't want to socialise for fear of eating 'bad' food.** If you don't want to go to your friend's birthday dinner because of the food that will be there, then it's a good idea to talk to someone—a family member, a friend or someone else you trust—about how you're feeling.

♡ **You place your worth in how much you weigh.** This is obviously ridiculous, but it happens all the time. Your weight has nothing to do with how amazing you are as a person, or whether people want to be around you or not. We are all different, and that's what makes us special. It's important to always remember that!

HEALTH, I BELIEVE,
IS ABOUT BEING THE BEST
VERSION OF YOURSELF
THAT YOU CAN POSSIBLY BE.
FOR ME, NUTRITION PLAYS
A HUGE PART IN THAT.

This was a turning point for me: I realised that I needed to do something to fix my mindset and my happiness. First thing was giving up on 'dieting', as it obviously wasn't working for me. I changed tack and, instead of counting calories, I simply started to eat when I was hungry and I ate what I wanted (all things in moderation), but tried to make healthier choices when I could. The change was self-evident! Almost immediately I stopped thinking about food all the time, I became much more social again, I felt far happier and I exercised when I felt like it rather than when I thought I should.

Also, once I stopped counting calories, I got better and better at making healthy choices when it came to food. Now it is mostly second nature, as I know how I feel when I eat nutrient-dense wholefoods—I have much more energy, can focus, and am far more positive overall. The trick is to find the right balance. You need to listen to your body and find the sweet spot where your body is fit and happy, and can sustain that certain weight long term.

The reason I share all of this with you is to show that health is about so much more than going to the gym or about what you do (or don't) eat. Health, I believe, is about being the best version of yourself that you can possibly be. For me, nutrition plays a huge part in that. These days, I try to eat as naturally as I can (with treats whenever I feel like them), and I can honestly say that doing so has contributed to me being happier, having more energy and generally feeling bloody awesome.

LAZY-GIRL PALEO

After the nutritional ups and downs of my younger years, I now consider myself a healthy, balanced eater. I follow a mostly paleo lifestyle, but I am pretty relaxed about it. Paleo comes from the term 'Paleolithic', which refers to the cultural period of the Stone Age that began about two and a half million years ago and is marked by the earliest use of tools made of chipped stone. The Paleolithic period ended at different times in different parts of the world—generally around 10,000 years ago in Europe and the Middle East—and is also sometimes called the Old Stone Age.

The paleo diet is centred on what humans are thought to have eaten in those days: meat, fish, eggs, fruit, veges, nuts and seeds. (I'm not sure that they ate camembert or chocolate back then, but I tell myself they did.) Personally, I believe that the paleo diet is

'Unreal' food

These days, so much of our food is loaded with artificial sweeteners and colours, and even many of our crops are sprayed with nasty chemicals. It can be next to impossible to live a life free of not-nice chemicals, but I believe it's important to try to limit them where possible by eating natural wholefoods that are organic and spray-free, and by trying to use all-natural skincare and household cleaning products where possible.

Fun fact: did you know that some research has suggested that 60 per cent of what we put on our skin ends up in our bloodstream? I don't know about you, but that scares the bejeezus out of me! Next time you're in the shower, take a look at the ingredients in your shampoo or body wash, and see if you can figure out what they actually are. If it looks like a bunch of mumbo-jumbo, it might be worth asking yourself, *Do I really want that stuff to end up in my bloodstream if I can't even pronounce it?* (You can read more about the all-natural skin products I like to use on page 167.)

Choose natural wherever possible—in your food and in the rest of your life!

the best framework for a healthy lifestyle, but that is only my opinion. What works for me may not work for someone else.

The hardest part about healthy eating is, I believe, starting. It can be tricky even knowing *where* to start. It's best to do your own research, try a few things and find what works best for your body. At the end of the day, we're all only human, and we're all doing our best. It might take you some time, but you just need to find the right balance for you when it comes to what you eat—whatever it is that you feel is achievable to make you feel good for the rest of your life. I find it works for me to take a '90 per cent of the time' approach, so that the remaining 10 per cent of the time I just eat whatever I want (a choc-top ice cream at the movies, obviously).

I try to centre all of my meals around natural, unprocessed foods. A little tip that someone once told me is to shop on the outer edge of the supermarket, as that's where all the fresh food lives—the theory being that the human body doesn't need anything that comes packaged. When I began eating mostly natural wholefoods, I started to have so much more energy, felt happier and slept better. I found myself wanting to eat crappy food less and less. Now I don't even really think about eating healthily (unless I've had a big week of over-indulging, then I try to stick to good, natural food a little more to give my body a bit of TLC).

However, I have to be very clear: I'm

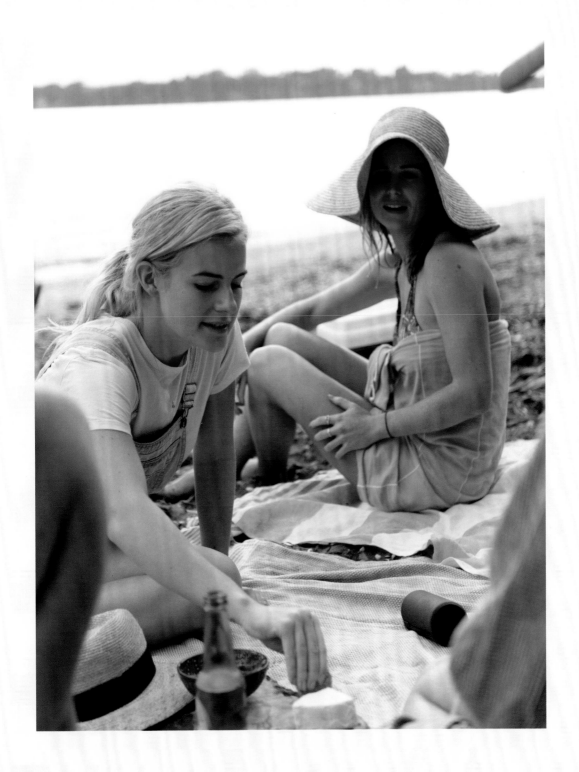

not talking about anything drastic. My approach to what I eat these days pretty much consists of minimising refined sugar and anything processed—it's really as simple as paleo pie! I do still eat a little bit of dairy, because I live for cheese and cream.

Of course, with any 'diet' (and I use that term loosely) can come judgement. I will never quite understand why some people try to make others feel bad or embarrassed about making healthy choices about what they eat. I've worked in many office environments, and I couldn't tell you how many times I have pulled out a healthy lunch and someone has felt the need to say, 'Jeez, *that's* healthy! Body is a temple, is it?'

It always makes me feel slightly uncomfortable, even though I know it shouldn't! I find it hard to imagine anyone saying anything like that if it was the other way around—'Woah, *doughnut* for lunch? *Someone* doesn't care about their body!'—because that would just be mean. I can't work out why it's socially acceptable the other way around. I think deep down some people react this way because they might feel that your decision to eat healthily is in some way a hidden judgement of their own choices, especially if they're feeling a bit bad about eating something they think they shouldn't have. I guess if you find yourself facing this kind of judgement it's important to remind yourself why you're choosing to eat what you are. It's OK to stand by the fact that you want to look after your body. Just remember, it's their problem, not yours.

One of the main reasons I love eating predominantly paleo is that I can still have all the foods I love, simply by subbing out a few things for a healthier version. I'm a huge fan of making healthier versions of my favourite meals. The child who could not live without spaghetti bolognese is still inside me, and I would die without fries, so I just tweak the recipes for these things slightly to make them fit in with my lifestyle. For example, I replace spaghetti with zoodles (noodles made out of spiralised zucchini) and make fries using kumara instead of potato. I'm still not fond of salad—it's just too bland and boring—and it was one of my New Year's resolutions to stop putting it on my plate simply because I felt pressured to do so. If I'm going to eat a salad, I want it to be the king of all salads—hearty, meaty and tasty.

Happily for you, in the following pages I've included a list of my go-to favourite recipes that are both healthy *and* delicious. I promise you won't feel like you're eating rabbit food! Also I have to add that these are true lazy-girl recipes: quick, easy and with simple measurements.

That's what I'm all about! I hope you enjoy them.

A day in the diet of Matootles

The word 'diet' is a funny thing. For me, 'diet' just means the foods I like to eat, but it has somehow morphed into this idea of eating a certain way to lose weight—and that kind of diet is often not sustainable in the long term. In this sense, paleo for me is more of a lifestyle than a diet, I guess. I think of paleo as a nutritional framework that I choose to follow as much as possible because I find it makes me feel the best and gives me a whole bunch of energy. (I don't even need coffee any more!)

I'm a huge advocate of a balanced approach when it comes to food, but the following is an example of what a typical day might look like for me (and my belly).

- ♡ **Breakfast:** my Chocolatey Dream Smoothie (see recipe on page 88).
- ♡ **Lunch:** fried eggs and smashed avocado on paleo toast (or with some bacon, if I don't have the bread).
- ♡ **Dinner:** barbecued steak with home-made Kumara Fries (see recipe on page 118) and steamed broccoli drizzled with olive oil and lemon.

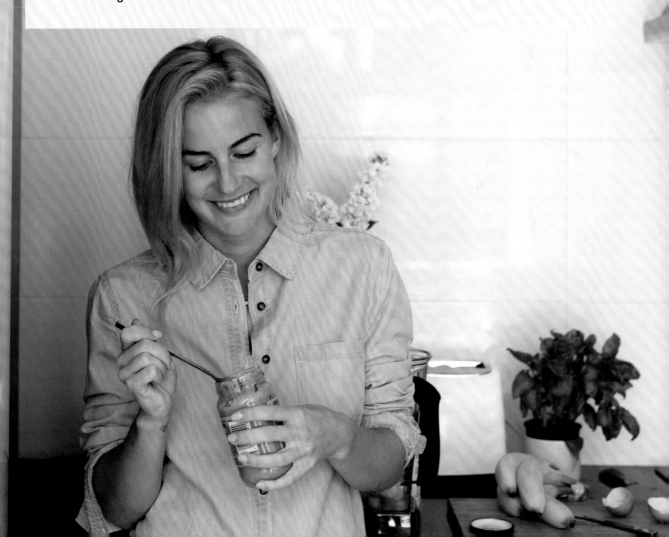

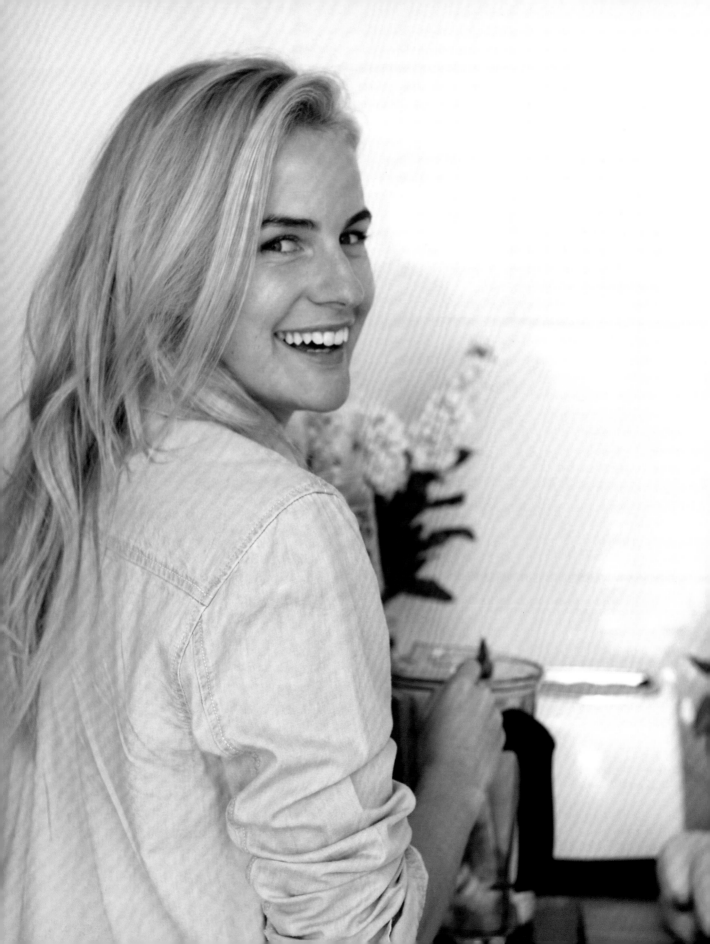

RECIPES

CHOCOLATEY DREAM SMOOTHIE

Serves 2

You may have seen this recipe on my blog, but I have it most days so it seems a crime to not share it in this book too. If you have a bit of a sweet tooth like I do this completely satisfies it without the need for chocolate (although obviously I still have that now and again). This one is packed with good fats, so it will fill you up for ages.

———————

1 banana
1 tablespoon peanut butter
small handful of spinach
¼ cup cacao powder
¼ cup CleanPaleo chocolate protein powder*
1 cup (250 ml) coconut milk**
2 free-range eggs
1 tablespoon pure maple syrup
half an avocado (optional, to make it creamier)
handful of ice

Put all your ingredients into a blender, then blend everything together well.

Pour into two glasses and enjoy!

———————

* *This may look like shameless promotion of my boyfriend's company, which it kind of is, but it is also the best protein powder for anyone who wants one that's natural and kind to your tummy. You can get CleanPaleo products at good food retailers, or online at clean-paleo.com.*

** *I use Little Island Coconut Milk for my smoothies, but you can use any milk you like—almond, cow, whatever . . .*

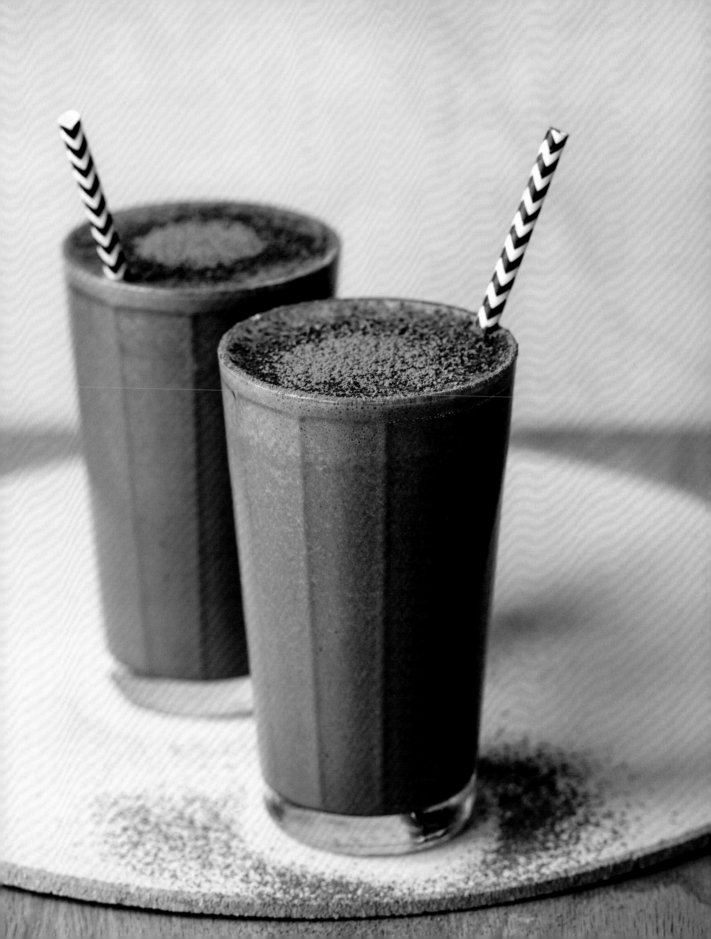

GREEN SMOOTHIE

Serves 1

Everyone needs a go-to green smoothie recipe. My inspiration and friend Ben Warren, a clinical nutritionist from BePure, recommends that you have leafy greens with every meal, every day. I try my darndest, but I don't often get there, so this super-quick, super-nutritious smoothie does the trick when I feel like I need an injection of greens.

---

handful of kale or spinach
2 whole kiwifruit, skin on and
  washed with water to remove
  any possible pesticides
juice of ½ lemon
1 free-range egg
pinch of cinnamon
½ teaspoon vanilla essence
1 tablespoon pure maple syrup
200 ml coconut milk

Put all your ingredients into a blender, then blend everything together well.

Pour into a glass and enjoy!

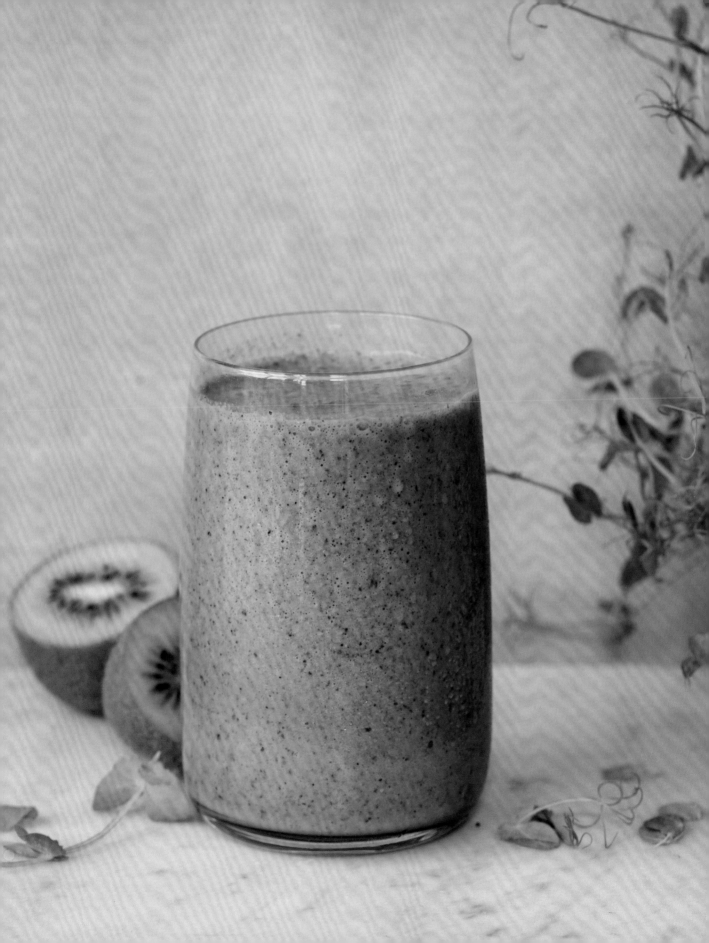

'I'M BERRY THIRSTY' SMOOTHIE

Serves 1

A great pun, if I do say so myself. This one definitely has a summer vibe. It makes me think of cocktails on the beach in Fiji, instead of sitting on my couch in my PJs scrolling through social media, which is 100 per cent what I do when I drink this.

---

handful of blueberries
handful of strawberries
handful of blackberries
½ cup (125 ml) coconut yoghurt
2 tablespoons CleanPaleo vanilla
   protein powder*
1 teaspoon vanilla essence
1 cup (250 ml) coconut milk

Put all your ingredients into a blender, then blend everything together well.

Pour into a glass and enjoy!

---

* *You can get CleanPaleo products at good food retailers, or online at clean-paleo.com.*

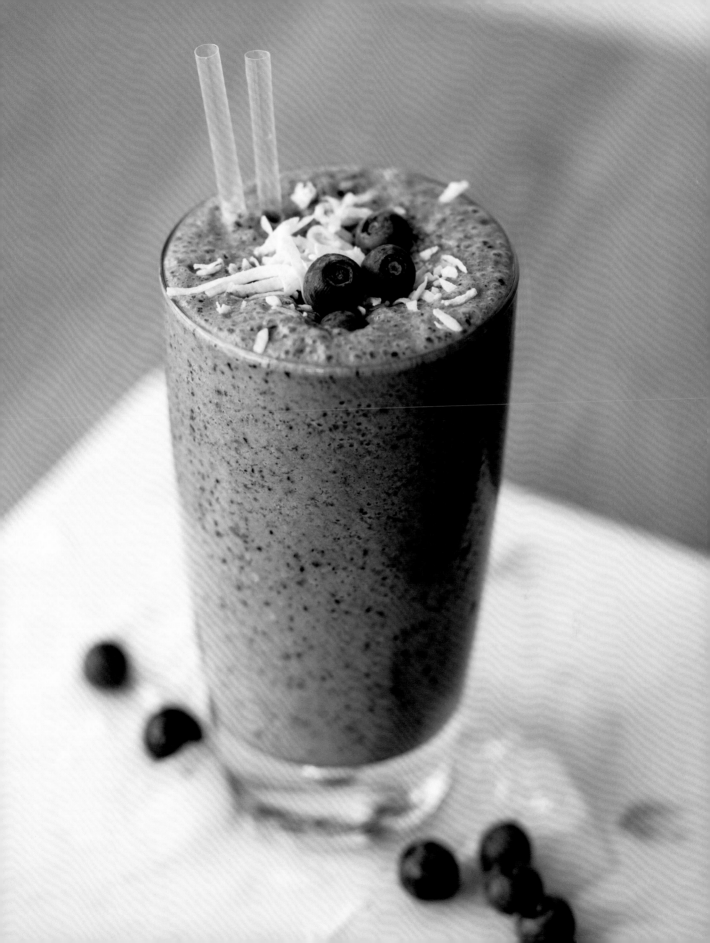

PALEO PORRIDGE

Serves 1

When I adopted a paleo lifestyle, one of the things I had to say goodbye to was porridge. I mean, it's literally a massive bowl of cereal grains . . . kind of goes against the whole paleo no-grain thing, right? So I decided I would create this version, which is just as delicious and fills me up more than the original. (OK, I lied. I didn't create it. Art did. But don't worry, I got his permission to include it!)

¾ cup CleanPaleo Original Crunch breakfast blend*

¼ cup chia seeds

¼ teaspoon salt

1 cup (250 ml) almond or coconut milk

2 tablespoons pure maple syrup

Put the CleanPaleo Original Crunch in a blender and blend until it's as fine as you can get it. It will start sticking together slightly.

Transfer the blended Original Crunch to a saucepan, and mix in the chia seeds and salt with a wooden spoon. Stir in the milk and maple syrup.

Put on the stovetop over medium heat, and simmer for about 5 minutes, until it turns thick and gluggy.

To serve, put in a bowl and top with whatever you like—cream, fruit, yoghurt, ham . . .

---

* You can get CleanPaleo products at good food retailers, or online at clean-paleo.com.

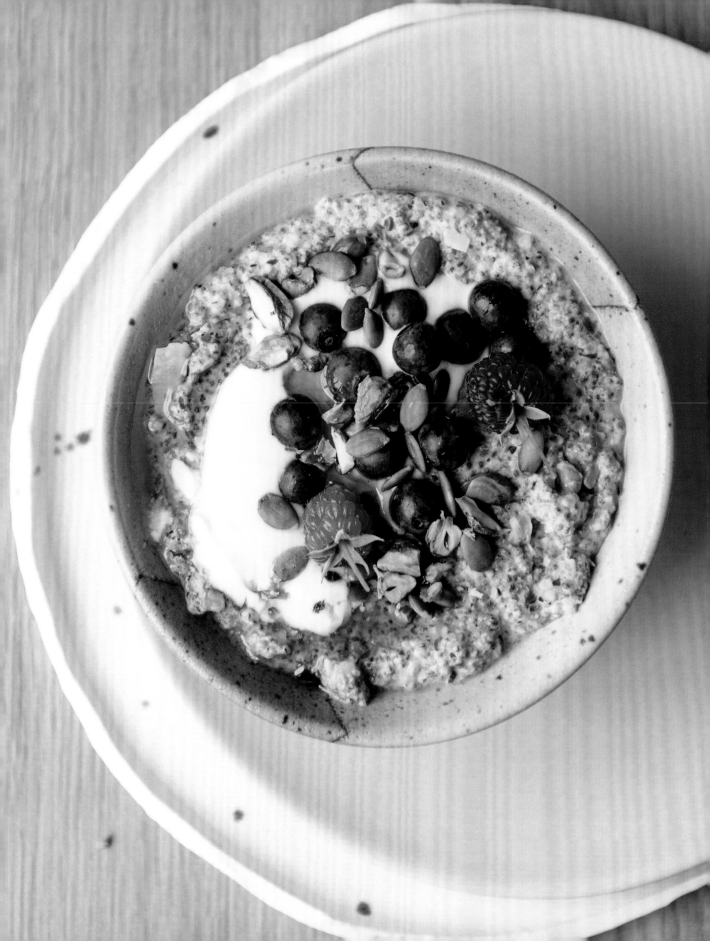

ULTIMATE OMMY

Serves 1

If you also follow a predominately paleo lifestyle, then I'm sure you eat a lot of eggs. If you're not careful, it's kind of easy to get sick of them (or for me it is, anyway). I'm always trying to find ways to dress my eggs up to make them a bit more exciting than just scrammys on toast. Ommys (omelettes) are a great way to do that, as they are so versatile (that's the beauty of them). You can use this recipe as a base and change the added ingredients for whatever you like, really—although I highly recommend keeping chorizo in there, as it's delicious.

---

3 large free-range eggs

salt and pepper, to taste

1 teaspoon butter

½ red onion, peeled and sliced into half moons

1 spicy Spanish chorizo sausage, sliced

3–4 slices tasty cheese

50 g ball (approx.) buffalo mozzarella, torn into pieces

In a small bowl, beat the eggs with the salt and pepper. Set aside.

Heat the butter in a frying pan over medium heat. Add the onions and cook, stirring occasionally, for about 4–5 minutes or until golden. Add the chorizo and cook, stirring occasionally, for a further 2 minutes.

Pour the eggs over the onion and chorizo, and gently stir to distribute the onions and chorizo evenly. Scatter the cheeses over the top. Cook for 2–3 minutes, until the bottom is starting to set. Using a wide spatula or fish slice, gently lift the omelette to allow the uncooked egg from the top to slide underneath, where it will cook faster.

Once the bottom is set and the top is looking nearly set—after another 3–4 minutes—use your spatula to fold the omelette in half. It will continue to cook while you get ready to move it to the plate.

To serve, transfer very carefully to your serving plate. Eat that ommy!

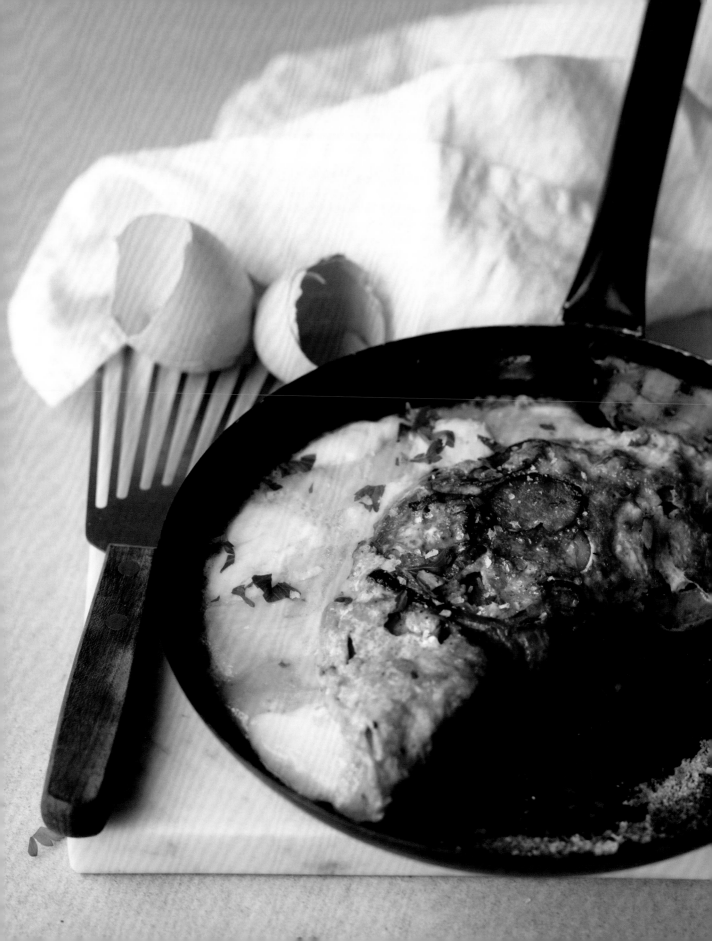

SPAGHETTI BOLOGNESE WITH ZOODLES

Serves 3–4

Mince is kind of my thing. It's literally my favourite food, and some mornings I wake up thinking about it. That's how much I love it. I grew up on spaghetti bolognese and it's a solid favourite of mine. Unfortunately, the usual wheat spaghetti doesn't quite fit with my paleo lifestyle, so I've tweaked things a tad to make it fit. There's no way I would ever get rid of spaghetti bolognese! My not-so-secret secret when it comes to making a good bolognese sauce is to let it simmer for a long time. I'm talking an hour, at least. It gives the flavours a chance to come out of their shells, and is the difference between an average mince dish and a magnificent mince dish.

4–5 zucchini, ends trimmed

dash of olive oil (or whatever oil you prefer)

1 brown onion, peeled and chopped

1 kg beef mince

1 x jar (approx. 500 g) good-quality, sugar-free, organic tomato pasta sauce

1 x 400 g can chopped tomatoes (one with basil included is good)

3 tablespoons tomato paste

handful of any fresh Italian herbs you can get, such as thyme, oregano or basil

2 tablespoons garlic powder

dash of chilli powder

dash of red wine (only if you're over eighteen, thank you very much)

shaved parmesan, to serve

Start by making your zoodles (see page 114). If you don't have a spiraliser (which you totally should, by the way, as they are AMAZING), then a julienne peeler will suffice. Put zoodles in a heatproof measuring jug or bowl and set aside.

Add the oil to a large frying pan, then sauté the onions over medium heat until they start to go clear. Add the mince, and sauté until browned—do this in two separate batches so the mince doesn't stew. Add your pasta sauce, chopped tomatoes and tomato paste. Sprinkle in all your herbs, garlic and chilli powders, and a little red wine (if using).

Reduce the heat, and let that baby simmer for at least an hour, stirring occasionally.

When you're ready to serve, cover your zoodles with boiling water. Leave them for about 5 minutes, then drain. Put the zoodles into a massive bowl, and pour the bolognese over the top. Scatter over parmesan and serve.

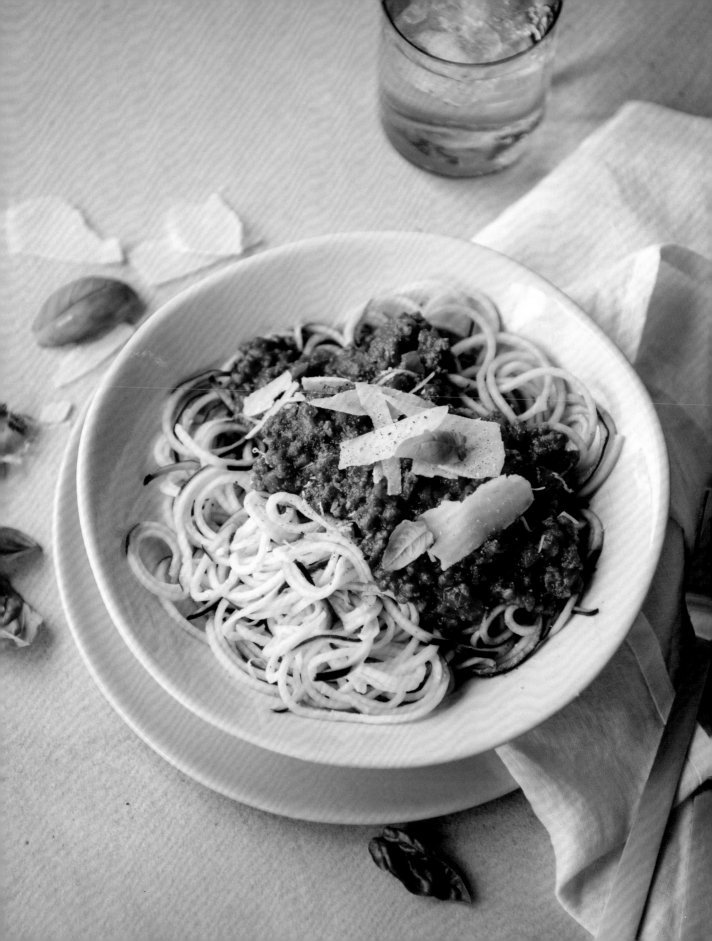

MEATZZA

Serves 4

Yeah, I wasn't lying when I said I was obsessed with mince. Pizza is another favourite of mine, so this is kind of like the love child of my two favourite foods. It's pretty meaty (as you may have guessed from the name), so I'd probably steer clear of it if you're a vegetarian.

---

1 kg beef mince
1 brown onion, peeled and chopped
1 clove garlic, peeled and crushed
1 free-range egg
handful of grated parmesan
salt and freshly ground black
    pepper, to taste
a few globs (about ½ cup) tomato
    paste
1 x 400 g can chopped tomatoes,
    drained
1 tablespoon olive oil
½ green capsicum, deseeded and
    sliced
½ red capsicum, deseeded and
    sliced
1 spring onion, green part only,
    chopped
handful of fresh basil leaves, plus
    extra to garnish
handful of fresh oregano leaves
50 g ball (approx.) buffalo
    mozzarella, torn into pieces
    (optional)

Preheat your oven to 210°C, and line a baking tray with baking paper.

In a large bowl, mix together the mince, onion, garlic, egg and parmesan, and season well with salt and pepper.

Place the meat on the prepared tray and, using wet hands, flatten it out as thinly as possible in a circle. Cover with cling film and use a rolling pin to roll it even thinner, so it's about 28–30 cm in diameter. Remove and discard the cling film.

Cook for 10 minutes, then remove from the oven.

Reduce the oven temperature to 175°C.

Spread the tomato paste over the meat.

Mix the canned tomatoes with the olive oil, then season with more salt and pepper, and spread over the tomato paste.

Top with the capsicum slices, spring onion and fresh herbs. Scatter over the pieces of buffalo mozzarella (if using), and return to the oven for a further 10 minutes, until the cheese has melted.

Garnish with fresh basil leaves and enjoy!

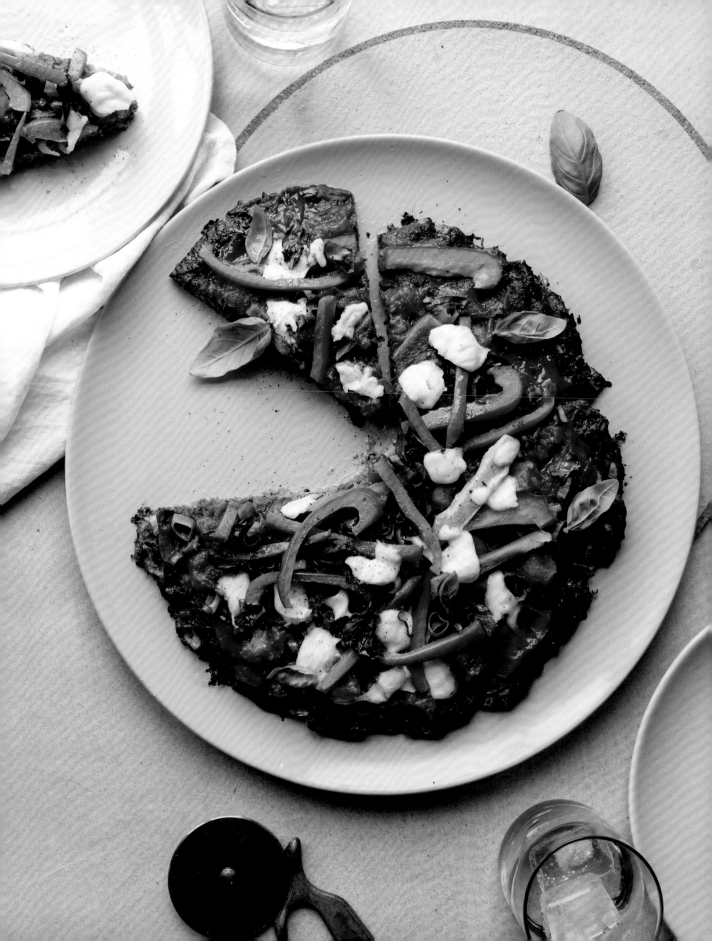

CHICKEN STIR-FRY LETTUCE CUPS

Serves 4

If you're anything like me and sometimes feel like your body just needs an injection of vegetables when you're a bit run-down, then you will love this recipe! It's super nutritious, packed with flavour and also pretty cheap to make. I make it all the time when I'm feeling lazy, as the vegetables can be changed out for whatever you have in the house.

---

1 head broccoli, cut into small florets

2 carrots, peeled and chopped

dash of olive oil

1 brown onion, peeled and chopped

3 cloves garlic, peeled and finely chopped (or lots of garlic powder if you can't be bothered)

500 g free-range, boneless, skinless chicken breast, finely chopped (or chicken mince)

2 teaspoons grated fresh ginger

3–4 tablespoons coconut aminos* or soy sauce

3–4 tablespoons sesame oil

1 red capsicum, deseeded and chopped

1 green capsicum, deseeded and chopped (or yellow if you're into it; I don't discriminate)

1 iceberg lettuce, leaves separated and washed

sesame seeds, to serve

Bring a pot of water to the boil, then add the broccoli and carrots. Boil for about 4 minutes, then drain and set aside.

Meanwhile, heat the olive oil in a saucepan, then add the onion and garlic and sauté until the onion starts to shine. Add the chicken and sauté until it is cooked through. Add the ginger, coconut aminos or soy sauce and sesame oil, and stir. Add the capsicum, and cook until soft—or, if you prefer to keep it crunchy, don't sauté it for too long. Add the broccoli and carrots, and mix everything carefully together.

Serve in the iceberg lettuce leaves, and sprinkle with sesame seeds if you want to look profesh.

---

* Coconut aminos is a sauce made from coconut sap that you can use instead of soy sauce. (Unlike soy sauce, it's paleo friendly.) You can find it at good food retailers or online.

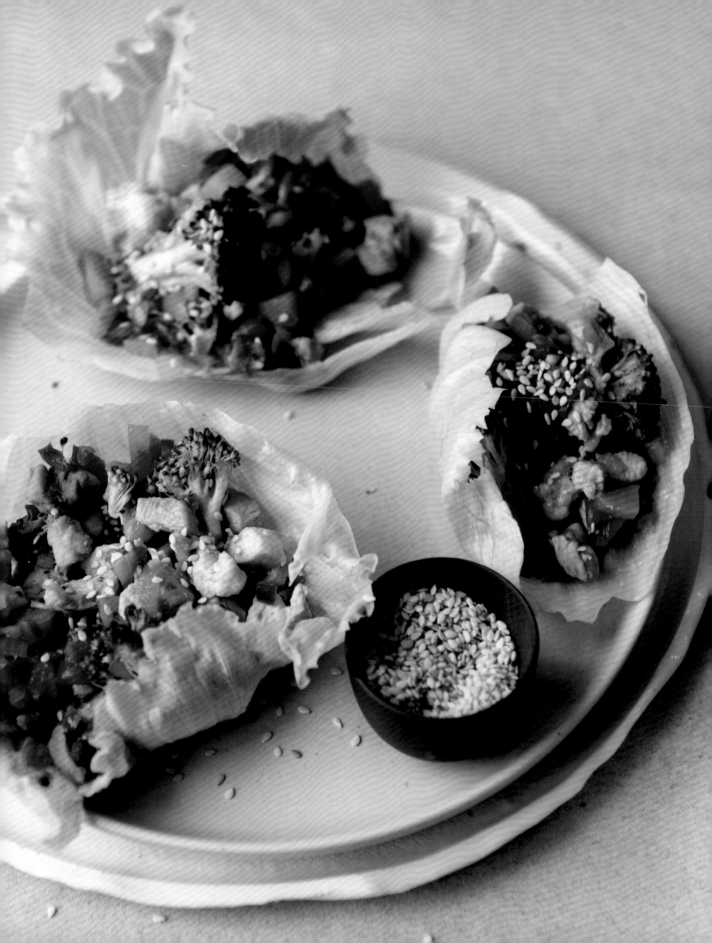

'LETTUCE EAT!' BURGERS

Serves 4

See what I did with the name there? I'm pretty sure it's been done before, but I like to think I made it up. Home-made burgers are great for when you have people round for a casual dinner, as all you really need to do is chop up the ingredients then serve all the bits individually and let people make their own burgers. It definitely saves a lot of faffing about. I guess I should note that lettuce burgers can get pretty messy (since there's no bun to absorb the meat juice), so use napkins and be prepared to get your hands a little dirty. My Kumara Fries (see page 118) are the perfect accompaniment to these burgers.

Spice mix

1 teaspoon ground cumin

1 teaspoon garlic powder

1 teaspoon paprika

salt and pepper, to taste

1 teaspoon onion powder (if you can find it—it's like gold!—otherwise just leave it out)

pinch of cayenne pepper

pinch of dried thyme

Burgers

1 kg beef mince

1 brown onion, peeled and chopped very finely

½ cup chopped spring onion

2 tablespoons cooking oil

1 iceberg lettuce, leaves separated and washed

your choice of fillings

your choice of sauce(s), such as aioli, tomato, chipotle or barbecue

To make the spice mix, put all the ingredients in a small mixing bowl and mix until well combined. Set aside.

To make the burger patties, in a large mixing bowl, combine the beef mince, brown onion and spring onion, then add the spice mix. With clean hands, mix until well combined. Shape into four balls. Flatten the balls into patties about 3 cm thick, then set aside.

Heat the oil in a frying pan over medium-high heat for 3–4 minutes.

Place the patties in the frying pan and cook for 4–5 minutes, until well browned. Flip and repeat on the other side. Remove from the pan and set aside.

To serve, put a burger pattie on a lettuce leaf, add your preferred fillings and sauces, then wrap everything up in the lettuce leaf. The options are endless for fillings— I usually have roasted red peppers, jalapeños and sliced avocado with mine.

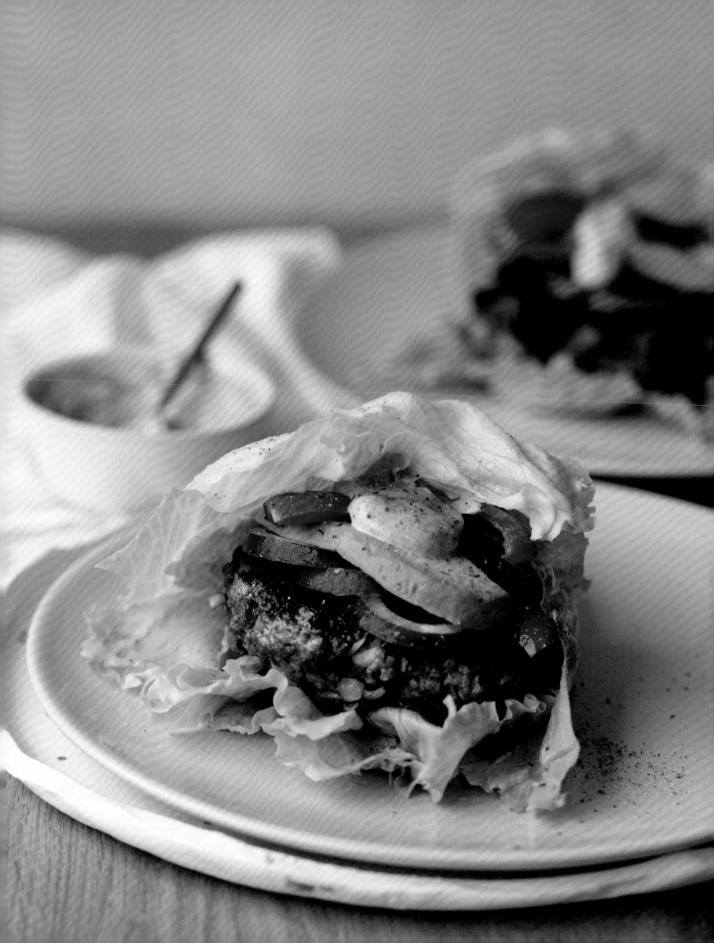

ZUCCHINI RAVIOLI

Serves 4

This one is really fun to make, and equally as delicious. It can be a bit fiddly to roll up the ravioli, so make sure you've given yourself a little bit of time. It can also look a bit gloppy at the end, but it's *so good* that you won't even care. You can keep it vegetarian, or you can add in some chicken if you just can't bear the thought of not having meat for dinner.

---

4 zucchini
2 cups (460 g) ricotta cheese
½ cup finely grated parmesan, plus
    extra to garnish
1 free-range egg, lightly beaten
1 garlic clove, peeled and finely
    chopped
handful of chopped basil
salt and pepper, to taste
1 x jar (approx. 500 g) good-quality,
    sugar-free, organic tomato pasta
    sauce
½ cup shredded mozzarella

Preheat the oven to 180°C, and grease a large baking dish with olive oil or butter.

First, make your zoodle strips. Slice the ends off each zucchini to create two flat ends. Using a vegetable peeler, peel each zucchini lengthwise into about 24 long, thin, flat strips. Keep peeling until you reach the centre of the zucchini. These are your 'pasta sheets', and they need to be as thick and wide as possible, so make sure you press reasonably firmly when peeling them.

Now make the filling. Combine the ricotta, parmesan, egg, garlic and basil in a medium-sized bowl. Season to taste.

Assemble the ravioli—this is definitely the fun bit! Lay out two strips of zucchini on a clean surface so that they overlap lengthwise, making a cross. Spoon about a tablespoon of filling into the centre of the cross. Bring the ends of the strips together to fold over the centre, one side at a time. Turn the ravioli over and place in the baking dish, seam-side down. Repeat with the remaining zucchini and filling—you should end up with about 12 parcels.

Pour the pasta sauce around the ravioli, and top with mozzarella and parmesan.

Bake for about 20 minutes, until the zoodles are al dente (cooked but still firm to the bite) and the cheese is melted and golden.

Serve with a simple side salad.

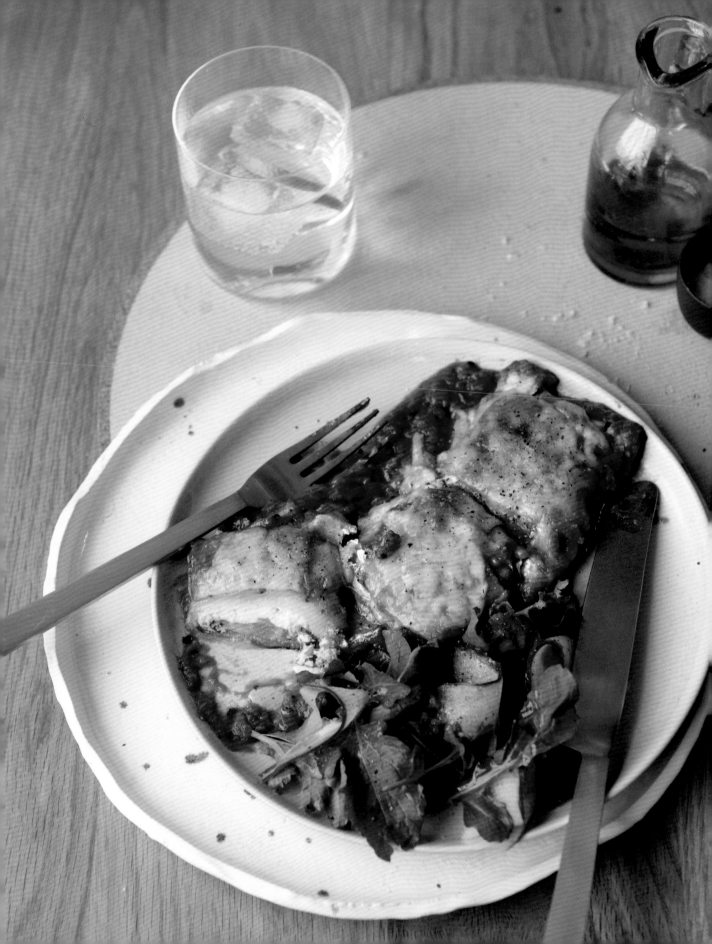

THAI GREEN CHICKEN CURRY

Serves 4

Who doesn't love a good curry? Curry makes me think of winter nights and snuggling up in front of the telly (or Netflix). Coconut milk is the base for this dish, so it's filled with healthy fats and is really filling. As my Dad says, 'It's just like a bought one!' If it's not spicy enough for you (I'm a little bit of a wuss when it comes to spice), then feel free to add some fresh chilli as well. Oh, and a little tip: don't tell people you used curry paste and they will think you're a culinary genius.

---

1 tablespoon coconut oil

2 medium shallots (or 1 large brown onion), peeled and chopped

3 cloves garlic, peeled and chopped

1 teaspoon grated fresh ginger

2 tablespoons green curry paste (try to find one with little or no added sugar)

1 x 400 ml can full-fat coconut milk

4 carrots, peeled into ribbons

2 teaspoons gluten-free fish sauce

2 tablespoons coconut aminos*

1 zucchini, cut into 1 cm slices

1 kg free-range, boneless, skinless chicken breasts, cut into thin strips

In a wok (I love using a wok) or a saucepan with high sides, heat the coconut oil over medium-high heat. Add the shallots, and cook briefly until shiny and see-through. Add the garlic and ginger, and cook for about a minute. Add the curry paste, coconut milk, carrots, fish sauce and coconut aminos. Simmer, uncovered, for 5 minutes, until the carrots begin to soften.

Add the zucchini, and simmer for a couple of minutes. Add the chicken, and simmer for another 5–7 minutes, until the chicken is just cooked and the vegetables are tender. Serve in bowls with cauliflower rice (see page 110).

---

* Coconut aminos is a sauce made from coconut sap that you can use instead of soy sauce. (Unlike soy sauce, it's paleo friendly.) You can find it at good food retailers or online.

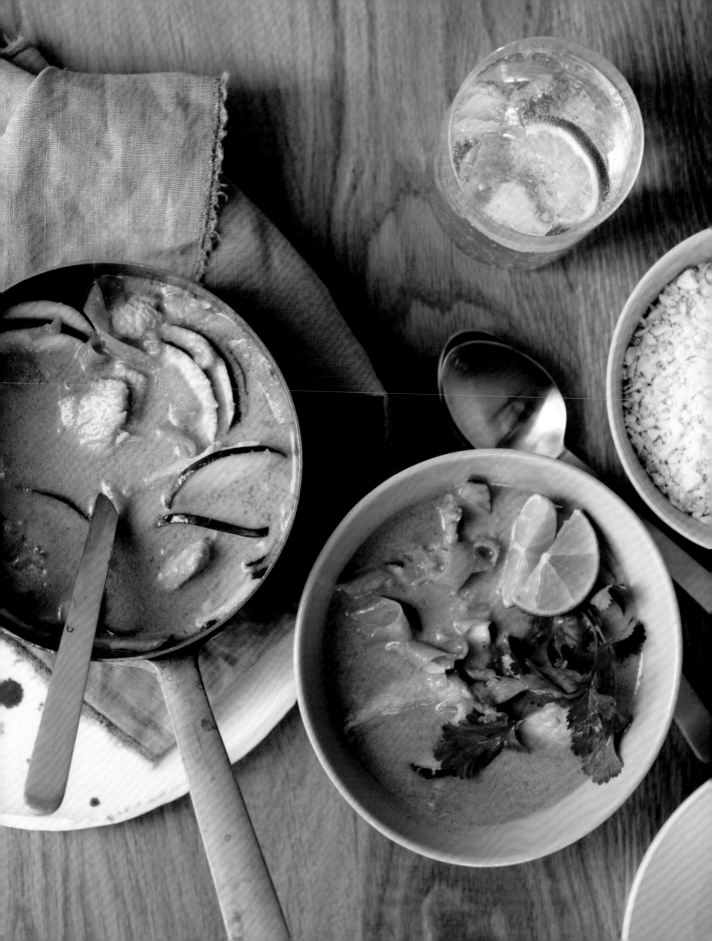

CHILLI CON CARNE WITH CAULIFLOWER RICE

Serves 4

Just the thought of this dish makes me feel all warm inside. It's the perfect comfort food for the winter months and is pretty much a weekly staple for me when it's cold. I was inspired by Jamie Oliver when I came up with this chilli recipe back when I was living in London, where the winters were seriously intense. In Jamie's version, he melts in a piece of dark chocolate. I've done it once, and to be honest I could hardly taste it, but give it a go and see what you think!

---

2 tablespoons olive oil (or whatever oil you prefer)

1 kg beef mince

2 brown onions, peeled and chopped

2 cloves garlic, peeled and finely chopped

2 carrots, peeled and chopped

2 red capsicums, deseeded and roughly chopped

2 sticks celery (not essential if you hate celery)

1 heaped teaspoon chilli powder

1 heaped teaspoon ground cumin

1 heaped teaspoon ground cinnamon

sea salt and black pepper, to taste

1 x 400 g can chickpeas, drained (optional)

1 x 400 g can red kidney beans, drained

2 x 400 g can chopped tomatoes (ideally including herbs)

small handful fresh coriander

2 tablespoons balsamic vinegar

1 head cauliflower

lime wedges, to serve (optional)

Heat 1 tablespoon of oil in a large lidded saucepan over medium-high heat. Add the mince, and sauté until browned. Remove from the pan and set aside.

Add the chopped veges, the spices and a good pinch of salt and black pepper to the pan, and cook for 7 minutes, or until softened, stirring regularly.

Add the chickpeas (if using) and kidney beans. Tip in the tomatoes, then pour in a can's worth of water.

Pick the coriander leaves and set aside. Finely chop the stalks and add to the pan, along with the balsamic vinegar. Bring to the boil, then reduce the heat to low and simmer, covered with a lid, for at least an hour, or until slightly thickened and reduced, stirring occasionally.

Meanwhile, chop up the cauliflower, and remove and discard any big stalky bits. Place the chopped cauliflower in a food processor and pulse until it is the size of rice grains. If you don't have a food processor, never fear! Just grate the cauliflower with a cheese-grater.

Heat the other 1 tablespoon of oil in a frying pan over medium heat. Add the cauliflower rice, and season. Cover the frying pan and cook for about 3–5 minutes, until heated through. Fluff with a fork.

Divide rice and chilli between bowls, sprinkle with coriander leaves and serve with a lime wedge.

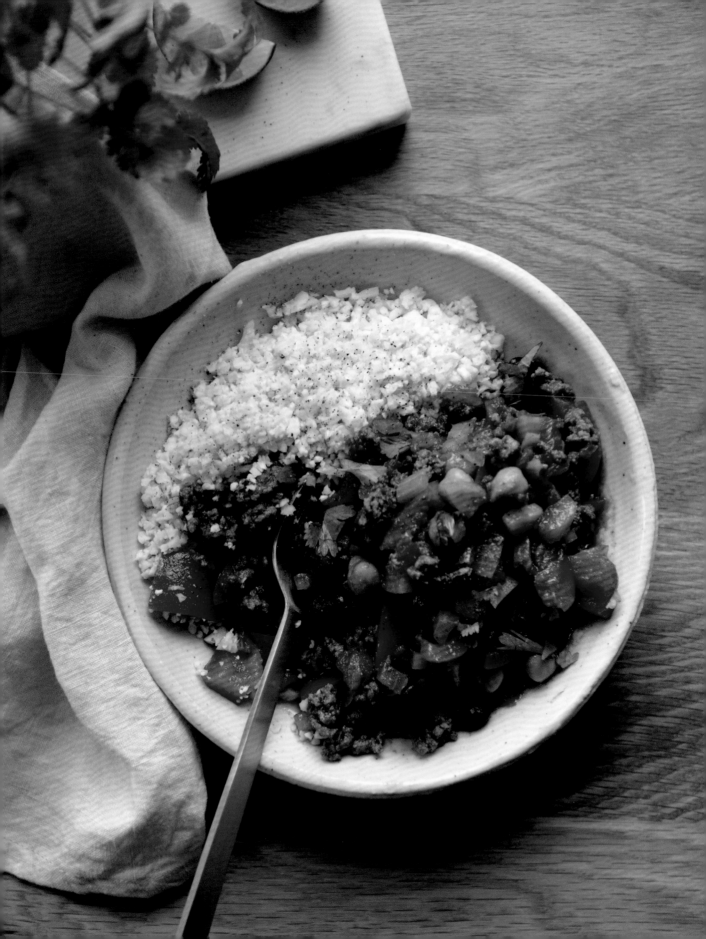

MEXICAN ZOODLE SOUP

Serves 2

I bloody love zoodles! They are such a great way to add some green veges to your meal when zucchini are in season without unnecessary expense and for getting the joy of noodles without the wheat. If you don't like spicy food, I would recommend going easy on the chilli powder. And maybe leave out the jalapeños—those bad boys are hot!

---

1 tablespoon olive oil

1 brown onion, peeled and chopped

4 garlic cloves, peeled and finely chopped

1–2 free-range, boneless, skinless chicken breasts, cut into cubes (or 2 x 400 g cans chickpeas, drained)

salt and pepper, to taste

2 teaspoons cumin

2 teaspoons chilli power

pinch of chipotle powder or cayenne pepper (depending on how much spice you can handle in your life)

1 teaspoon dried oregano (or a couple of bay leaves)

1 fresh tomato, chopped

1–2 tablespoons jalapeños, depending on how spicy you like it (optional)

4 cups (1 litre) chicken stock

4 cups (1 litre) water

4–5 zucchini

half a handful coriander leaves, roughly chopped, plus extra to garnish

juice of 1 lime

avocado slices, to garnish

In a large saucepan, heat the olive oil over medium heat. Add the onion and garlic, and sauté for 1–2 minutes, without browning. Add the chicken (or chickpeas) and sauté for 5–6 minutes, until the meat begins to brown, stirring often.

Season with salt and pepper, then add the spices and oregano, and cook for another minute. Add the tomato, jalapeños (if using), stock and water. Bring to the boil over high heat.

Meanwhile, make your zoodles. Slice the ends off each zucchini to create two flat ends. If you have a spiraliser, spiralise the zucchinis. If you don't have a spiraliser, then a julienne peeler will suffice.

Once your soup is boiling, add the zoodles and most of the coriander. Bring back up to the boil, then reduce the heat to medium and simmer for about 5 minutes or so, or until the zoodles are done to your liking.

Squeeze in the lime juice, then taste and adjust the seasoning if necessary.

To serve, ladle into bowls and top with sliced avocado (if using) and extra coriander leaves. Slurp away and enjoy!

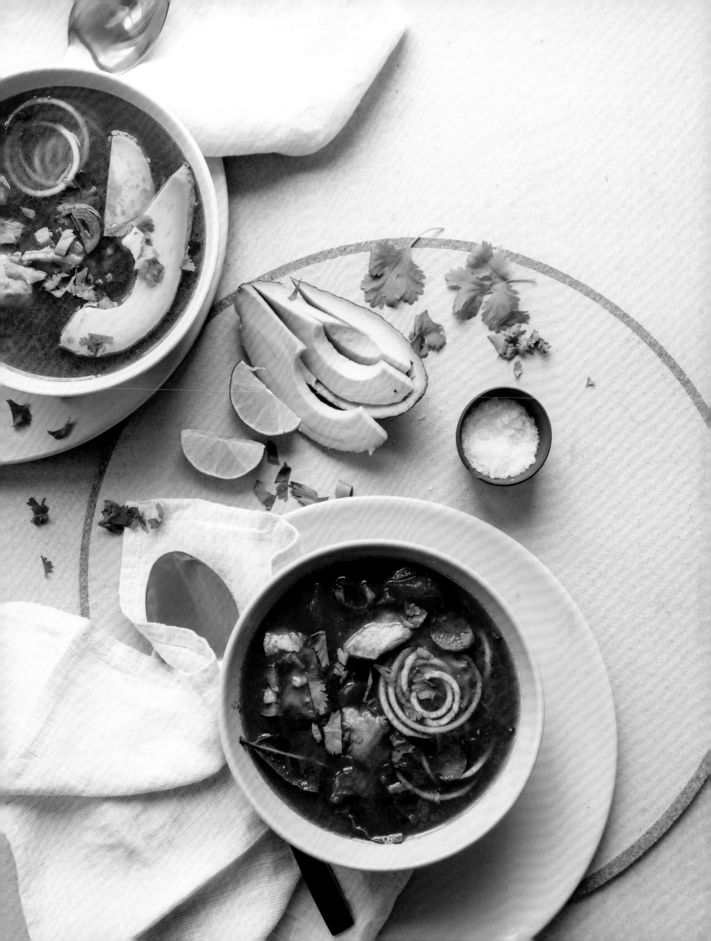

LAKSA

Serves 4

I love Asian food courts and I often find myself craving a really good laksa—but I
don't crave the sugar or additives that often come with the food-court versions.
This one here is all-natural and a definite crowd-pleaser, especially if you're trying
to impress someone in the ol' romance department. *Nudge, nudge.*

---

1 tablespoon olive oil

2 free-range, skinless, boneless
   chicken breasts, thinly sliced into
   bite-sized pieces

⅓ cup (60 g packet) laksa paste
   (try to find one with little or no
   added sugar)

4 cups (1 litre) chicken stock

1½ cups (375 ml) water

1 x 400 g can coconut cream

½ tablespoon fish sauce

4–5 zucchini

2 teaspoons coconut sugar
   (optional)

4 generous handfuls mung bean
   shoots (or substitute for any
   vegetables you want)

fresh coriander leaves, to garnish

sliced red chilli, to garnish

Heat the oil in a large saucepan over medium heat.
When the oil is hot, add the chicken and stir until
cooked. Add the laksa paste, and stir to coat the
chicken. Now add 1 cup (250 ml) chicken stock, and
stir until well combined. Add the remaining chicken
stock, water and coconut cream, and bring to the boil.
Reduce the heat, then add the fish sauce and simmer
for 10 minutes.

Meanwhile, make your zoodles. Slice the ends off each
zucchini to create two flat ends. If you have a spiraliser,
spiralise the zucchinis. If you don't have a spiraliser, then
a julienne peeler will suffice. Place your zoodles in a
large bowl and cover with boiling water. Leave them for
about 5 minutes, then drain.

Taste the laksa at this point, and add a little coconut
sugar if desired, or fish sauce if you like it a little more
salty. If the curry has thickened too much, you can thin
it with a little extra water.

To serve, divide zoodles among four soup bowls. Spoon
the laksa mixture over the top, then add a generous
handful of fresh bean shoots. Garnish with fresh
coriander leaves and sliced red chilli.

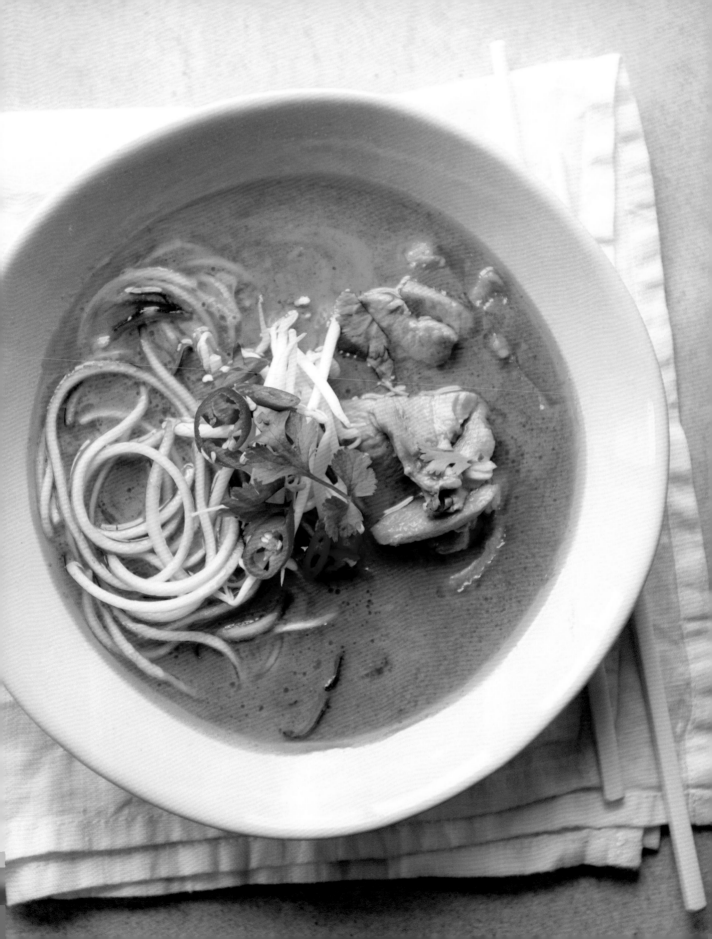

BEST ROAST VEGES YOU'LL EVER EAT

Serves 4

I have to give my dad, Ken Rice, a massive shout-out for this wee gem of a side dish. You know how dads tend to have a small repertoire of dishes, but that repertoire is damn good? That's what my dad is like. If you want a good pasta or a barbecue, Ken is your man. You can pretty much roast anything. If you decide to add any greens—you could add broccoli, green beans or anything—then maybe add them in halfway through, as God forbid they should be overdone!

---

3 kumara (approx. 500 g), cut into large chunks (I like orange kumara, but you can use whichever type you prefer)

2 red onions, peeled and cut into quarters

2 red capsicums, deseeded and cut into strips

8–10 whole garlic cloves, peeled and chopped

2 carrots, peeled and cut into large sticks

2 tablespoons olive oil

1 tablespoon balsamic vinegar (optional)

handful of chopped parsley, to garnish

aioli, to serve (optional)

Preheat your oven to 180°C.

Put the kumara, onions, capsicums, garlic and carrots into a large baking dish, and drizzle with the olive oil and balsamic (if using).

Bake for 20–30 minutes, or until the red onion has started to char a bit.

To serve, garnish with parsley. Serve as a side dish with some protein. This also goes really well with aioli (as most things do).

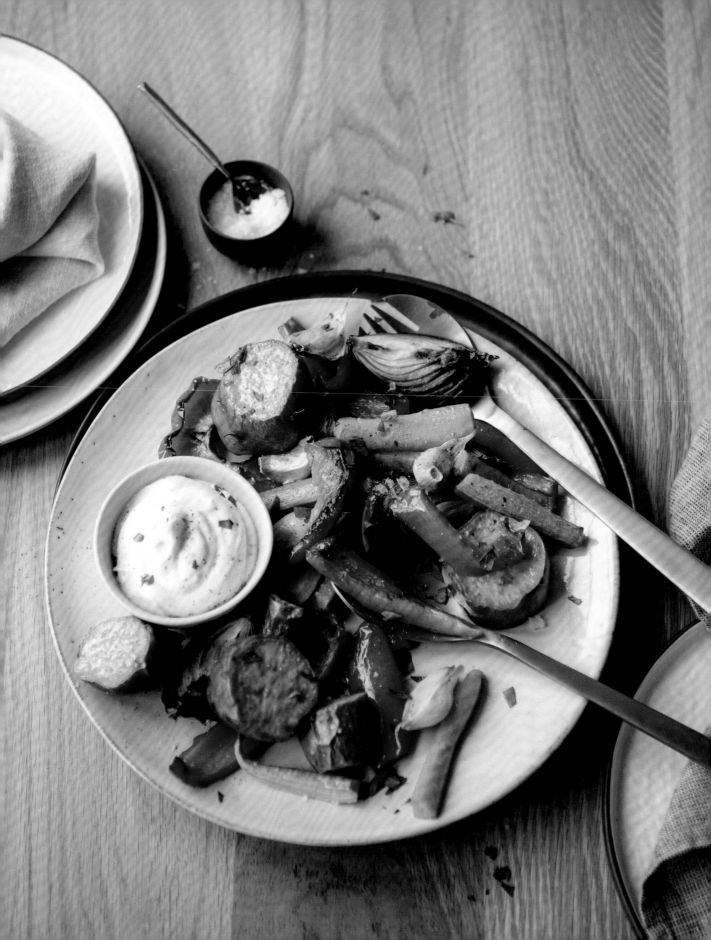

KUMARA FRIES

Serves 4

Do these even need an introduction? It's kumara in fries form, aka the *best* form. I actually have a deep-fryer at home, so I usually deep-fry these in olive oil, but this recipe doesn't need a deep-fryer and is just as good without. (I'm well aware that most people aren't so enthusiastic about kumara fries that they need their own deep-fryer.) The perfect accompaniment to pretty much anything, these are the goods. You can also have these with my Chilli con Carne (see page 110) to make chilli fries. You can use orange or purple kumara, but note that orange tends to come out softer.

3–4 kumara, skin on, scrubbed
    clean
2–3 tablespoons olive oil
pinch of cinnamon
dash of pure maple syrup
aioli, to serve

Preheat your oven to 180°C.

Cut the kumara into fries or wedges, and put into a large baking dish. Cover in the olive oil. Add the cinnamon and maple syrup and, using your hands, toss everything together so that all the fries are covered.

Bake for about 30 minutes, until slightly browned and crispy. Check on them while they're in the oven, and keep turning them so that they cook evenly.

Enjoy with some aioli on the side—and try not to eat all of them yourself.

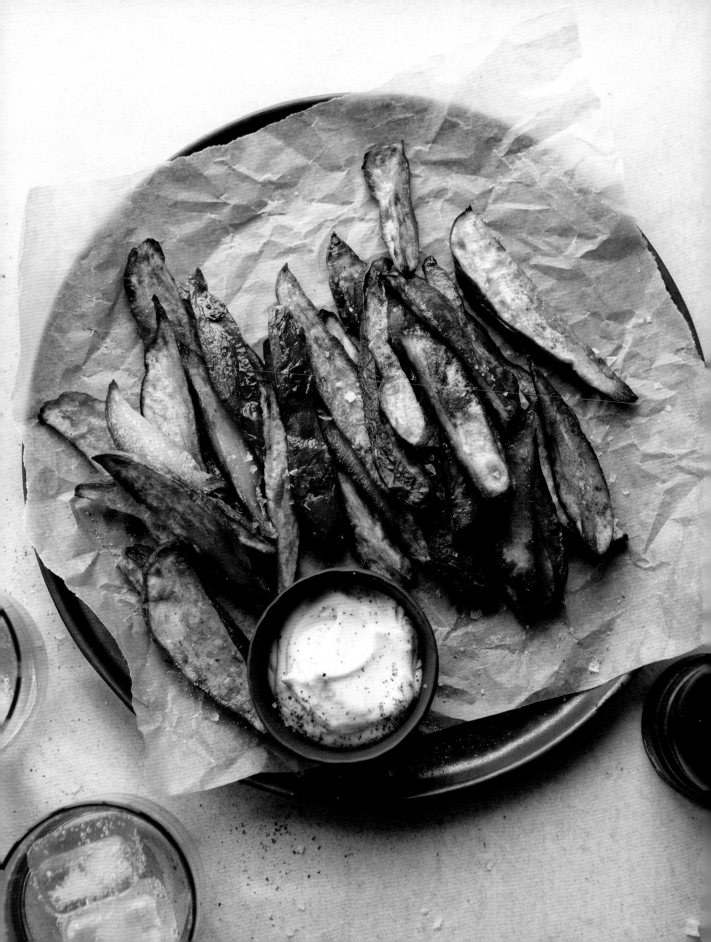

ALMOND BUTTER BROWNIES

Makes 12 squares

If you're going to a dinner party and you're on dessert, this is the perfect thing to make! It's super quick and also really nutritious, so if you're trying to make healthy choices it is a far better option than bringing along fruit. (Don't be that person.) If you don't want any refined sugar in there at all, you could take out the chocolate and substitute it for cacao nibs.

---

1 cup almond butter
¼ cup (60 ml) honey or pure maple syrup
¼ cup (60 ml) maple sugar or coconut sugar
1 free-range egg
1 teaspoon vanilla essence
½ teaspoon baking soda
pinch of sea salt
½ cup dark chocolate chips (or any chocolate you like, really)
cream or coconut yoghurt, to serve

Preheat oven to 180°C. Line a 20 cm x 20 cm baking tin with baking paper.

In a large bowl, mix together all of the ingredients except the chocolate chips and cream or yoghurt. Fold in the chocolate chips.

Pour the mixture into the prepared baking tin and spread out evenly. Bake for 15–20 minutes, then remove from the oven. The top will still seem a bit soft, but it will harden as it cools. Let cool in the tin for about 10 minutes before slicing.

Serve with cream or a dollop of coconut yoghurt alongside and you will think you're in heaven.

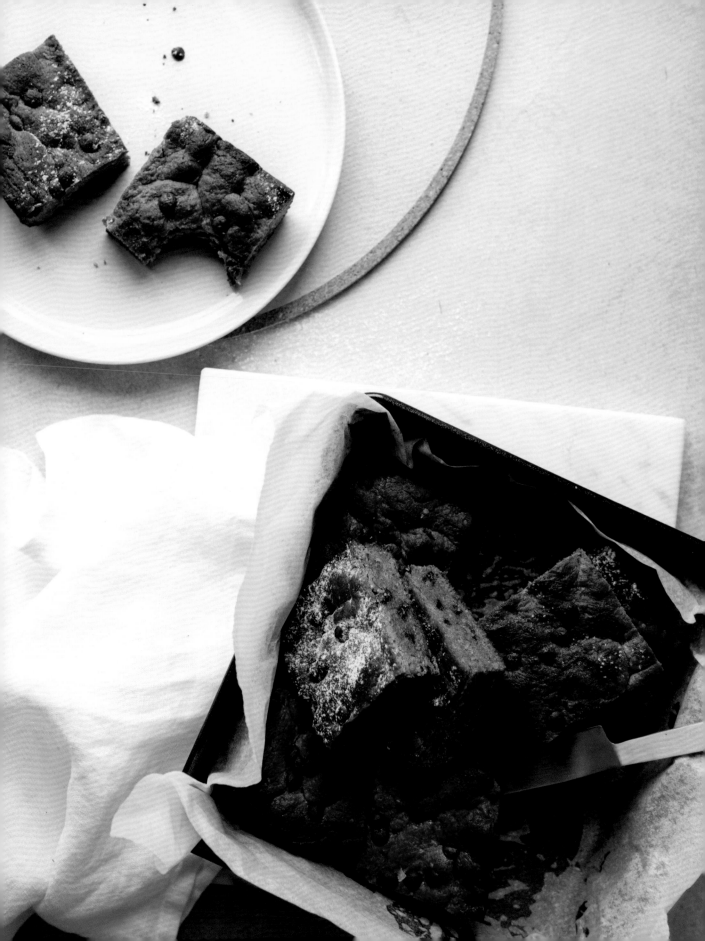

AVOCADO CHOCOLATE MOUSSE

Serves 3–4

The whole avocado-as-chocolate-mousse thing has really taken off in the last couple of years, so I'm sure this won't sound as disgusting to you as it did to me when I first heard about it. I had to make it for myself before I was really sure that it didn't feel like eating an avocado for dessert, and I promise you that you can hardly taste it! This is also a great, nutritious option to bring to a dinner party for dessert. Don't tell anyone it's avocado until they've finished. The reactions are hilarious.

---

200 g good-quality dark chocolate

2 ripe avocados, flesh chopped

½ cup (125 ml) almond or coconut milk

2 tablespoons honey or pure maple syrup (optional)

berries or any other fruit, to garnish (optional)

cacao powder, to garnish (if you're feeling crazy!)

Melt the chocolate in a double boiler or in a heatproof bowl set above a pot of simmering water. Make sure the water doesn't touch the bottom of the bowl, or the chocolate will burn and become grainy.

Pour the melted chocolate into the bowl of a food processor, add the avocado, and blend until smooth. Pour in the milk as you are blending. Keep blending until the mousse is very smooth and creamy. Taste, and if you would like it a little sweeter you can add a bit of honey or maple syrup.

Spoon into serving glasses or bowls, and chill in the fridge for 10–15 minutes before serving.

Garnish with fresh berries and a dusting of cacao powder, if you wish.

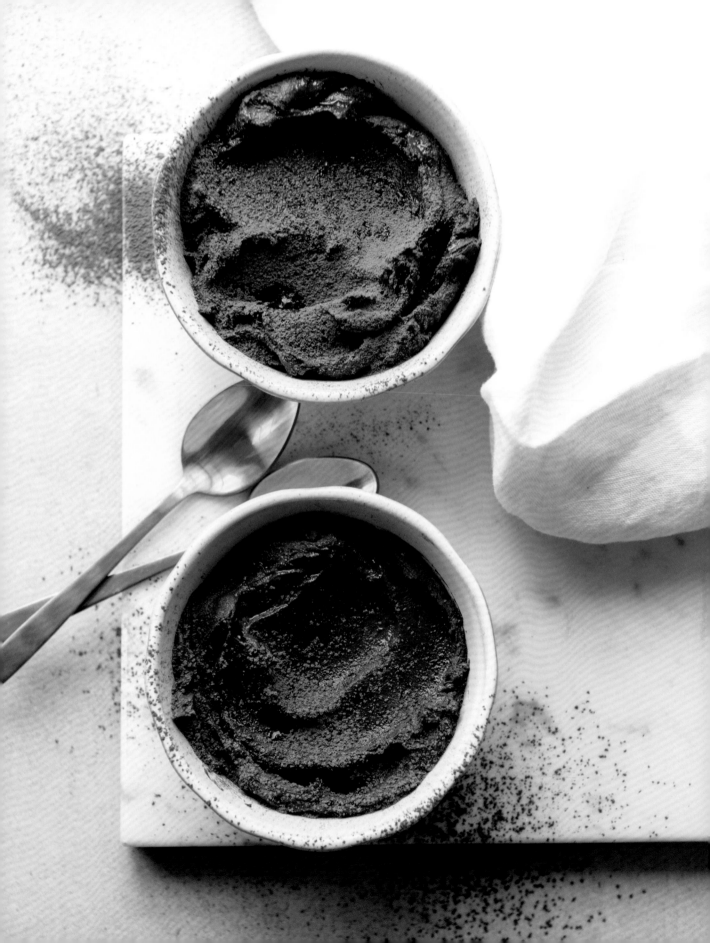

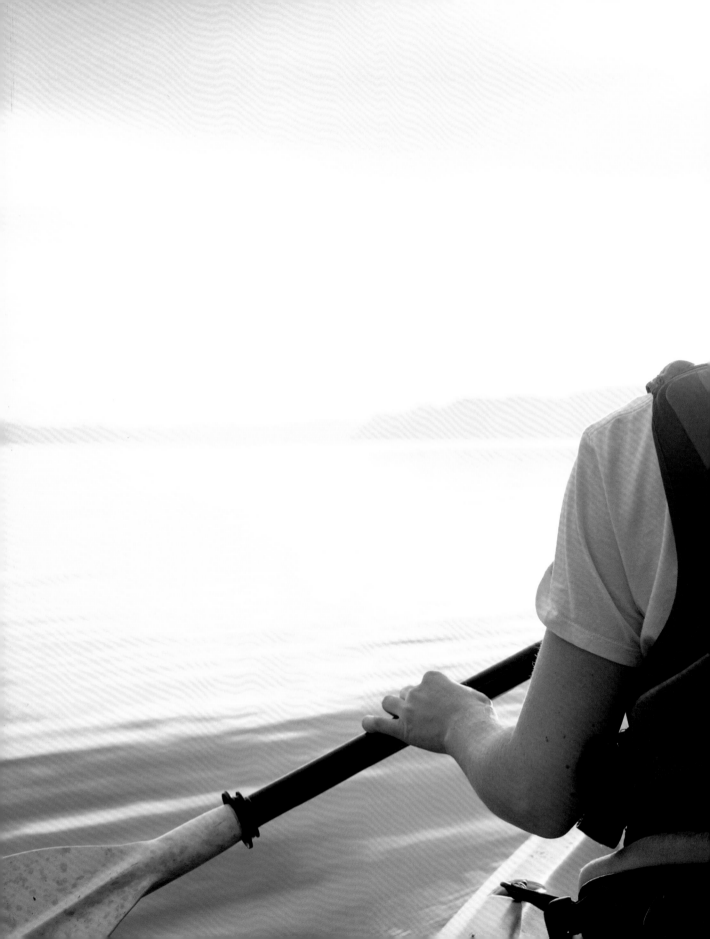

EXERCISE
AND FITNESS

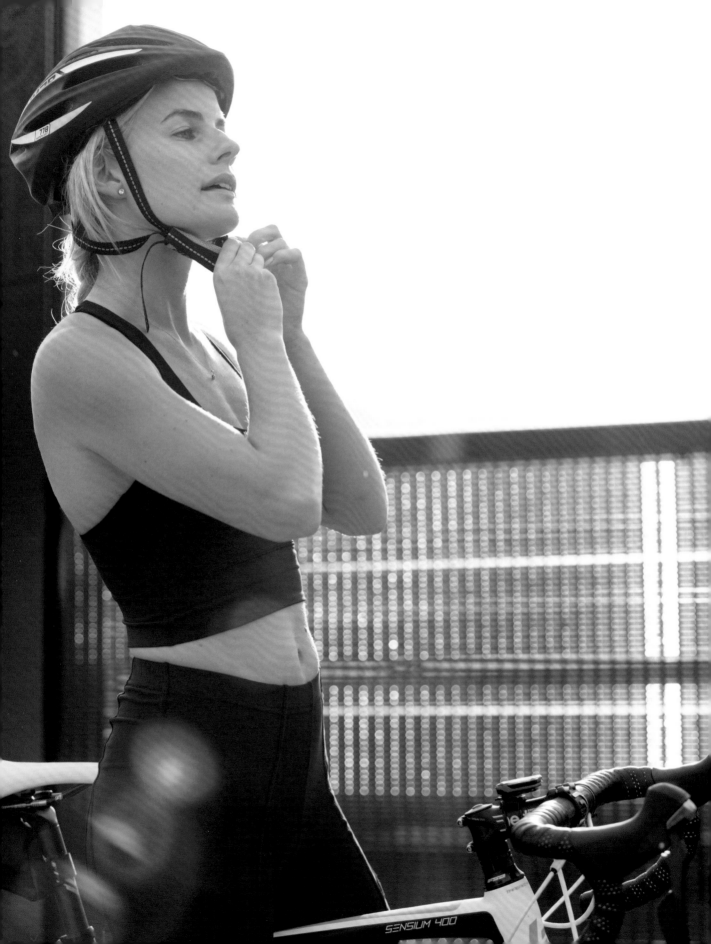

Ah, yes. Exercise. A lot of people have a love-hate relationship with exercise, and I totally get it. I have days when I set my alarm for 5.30 a.m. to get up for a workout . . . then end up hitting snooze until 7 a.m. For three days in a row.

Sometimes I'll wake up on a Saturday morning and get all dressed in my activewear with the best of intentions . . . then, before I know it, it's 8 p.m. and I'm eating butter chicken on the sofa and, even though I'm still wearing my activewear, I haven't done a single active thing.

I'm definitely not perfect. I go through stages of being really motivated, then I'll have patches where I'm not so much. But that's totally natural, so I don't beat myself up about it (and you shouldn't either). That said, I do understand the importance of getting your body to move. I always find it odd that people place far more emphasis on exercising their pets than they do on exercising themselves. We need exercise just as much as dogs do!

The average person needs at least an hour of light exercise a day—that includes walking, dancing, pole-dancing, whatever

Move your bum

I'm sure I don't need to tell most of you how good exercise is for you, but do you know exactly *how* good it is? I'm talking *really* good. Here's a quick run-down (excuse the pun) of the benefits of moving your bum.

♡ **It combats negative health conditions.** Regular exercise can help to prevent or manage a wide range of health problems and concerns, including stroke, metabolic syndrome, Type 2 diabetes, a number of cancers, arthritis, and even depression and anxiety.

♡ **It makes you happy!** Physical activity stimulates various brain chemicals that leave you feeling happier and more relaxed.

♡ **It gives you energy.** Once you start to increase the amount of exercise you do, you will find you have far more energy throughout the day, so you'll get more out of life and generally be more productive.

♡ **It's great for fat loss.** (If your goal is to get rid of some junk in the trunk.)

♡ **It helps you make friends!** A gym or sports team is a great way to meet new people, and even if you are a runner or a walker you can always do that with your mates.

you like doing that involves moving your body—or half an hour of high-intensity exercise a day, such as running, a gym class or a hard gym workout. I try to do at least half an hour a day, but sometimes I'll have weeks where I only exercise a couple of times because life takes over! When it does, don't beat yourself up about it. Just make sure you prioritise exercise, and get back into it when you can. Your body—and mind—will thank you for it.

DO WHAT YOU LOVE

Personally, I don't think you have to push yourself to your absolute limit at the gym and lift 100 kilos while grunting unnecessarily in order to get in shape. Obviously, it depends on your goals and what you enjoy doing, but if you want to fit exercise into your lifestyle forever then it needs to be enjoyable. It needs to be something you can sustain.

For example, if you hate running, don't force yourself to do it. You're not going to be able to keep it up for the rest of your life if you don't enjoy it. Although, when it comes to running in particular, I'd reserve making that decision until after you've run a few times and given your body a chance to build up some fitness. I won't lie to you: running is bloody hard when you're unfit. It sucks. But, as soon as you've got a reasonable level of fitness, it gets much easier—and much more enjoyable.

Little wins

Challenging yourself physically and mentally through exercise is so rewarding. When we are challenged, we are forced to motivate ourselves, and by facing challenges at every opportunity we experience these things I like to call 'little wins'—when you achieve something you thought you couldn't, no matter how small. There is no better feeling in the world than surprising yourself by doing something you never thought you could. It's important to acknowledge these little wins every time you experience one. When all of them add up, they make such a positive difference in your life.

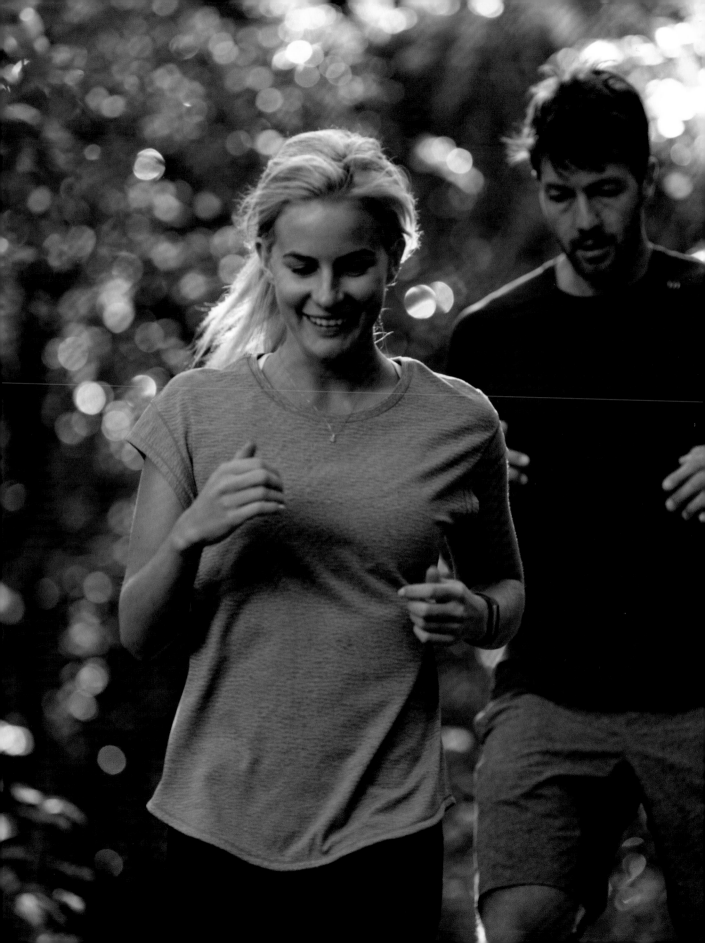

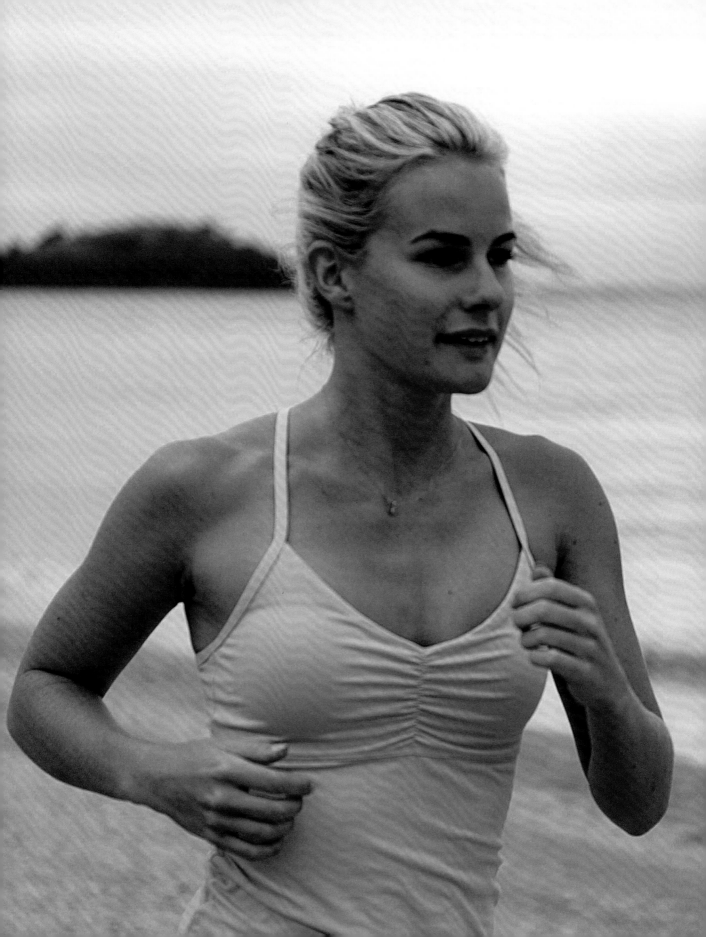

Four common fitness fibs

There's a whole bunch of opinions and theories out there when it comes to fitness, and now that we have 24/7 access to the interwebs it seems any Tom, Dick or Matootles can make something up and call it science. I don't know about you, but I find it incredibly frustrating trying to wade through everything to make sense of it all. So, to save you the pain, here are four common fitness fibs (adapted from a blog post I wrote a while back) debunked for your benefit.

1. **You can spot-reduce fat.** Sorry, guys. You can't choose where you lose weight. (I'm still upset about this one.) We're all different, and we all hold fat in different places. Your best shot is to focus on looking after yourself consistently, and on maintaining good overall health.

2. **The longer you work out, the more fat you burn.** This one is not 100 per cent true. Lazy girls, rejoice! A recent study published in the American College of Sports Medicine's *Health & Fitness Journal* concluded, 'A simple, fast, high-intensity workout—finished in as little as seven minutes—will produce many of the same benefits as a good run and trip to the weight room.' Furthermore, according to the Centers for Disease Control and Prevention, 'Several short workouts throughout the day are proven to be just as effective as one long-duration workout.'

3. **You have to lift!** Remember when Instagram first started and all of a sudden gajillions of fitness pages sprung up out of nowhere and everyone became obsessed with squats, deadlifts and lifting as heavy as possible at the gym? Yeah, I remember too—cos I was one of them! Of course, it totally depends on your goals, but I don't feel it's necessary to have veins popping out of your neck in order to get fit. These days I'm all about functional body-weight exercises, with a little cardio thrown in.

4. **If you're not sweating your ass off, you haven't worked hard enough.** I'm not convinced by this one, either. Sometimes I like a good sweat-a-thon, but a lot of the time I like to simply go for a walk, do yoga or do a light workout at the gym. I don't think there's anything wrong with that at all. As long as you're consistent with it, you will see results. They may be slower to come than if you sweated your ass off every day, but I'm OK with that.

—

A GREAT TIP FOR MAKING
EXERCISE ENJOYABLE
AND SUSTAINABLE IS TO
CONSTANTLY MIX IT UP, AND
TRY TO LIVE A GENERALLY
ACTIVE LIFESTYLE.

—

I used to hate running, but I love it now, especially because it's easy (kind of) and I can do it anywhere. All I need is my running gear and my shoes. I only discovered my love of running quite recently, when I entered the Auckland half-marathon. My training meant I had to run a few times a week for about three months in order to get to the fitness level I needed to be at. It was tough at first, as I had never really been a 'runner'. I hated it at the start—I couldn't even get to 2 kilometres without stopping—but by the end of it I loved the training, and was amazed at how far I had come in a few short months.

A great tip for making exercise enjoyable and sustainable (that sounds a bit environmental . . .) is to constantly mix it up, and try to live a generally active lifestyle. I've tried lots of different forms of exercise over the years, and now I dabble in a whole bunch of things so that I never get bored. Having a variety of options when it comes to exercise helps me with motivation, as I'm not doing the same thing over and over again.

Team sports are my favourite type of exercise as they kill two birds with one stone (though in no way do I condone actual killing of birds with stones): you can catch up with your friends and have a laugh, but also get a little workout in. If you're lacking in motivation, I highly recommend getting involved with a sports team. Playing sport socially is such a fun way to get moving, plus when you're committed to a team it's much harder to get out of it. I know that joining a social sports team can be pretty intimidating, but remember that people will respect you for getting involved and giving it a go. If you don't already know how to play, you will learn, and even slowly improve. I play in a social touch-rugby team every week, and I am by faaaar the worst player. I'm still not 100 per cent on all the rules (even though I've been in the team for two seasons now) and I drop the ball more than is considered acceptable, but I love it and my team is very supportive (luckily for me!). I'm still pretty rubbish, but I'm definitely less rubbish than when I joined the team, and that is a good feeling.

Aside from team sports and a bit of running here and there, I also do some at-home workouts (I'll take you through some of my favourites on pages 134–141), swim in the indoor pool if it's raining outside, and just recently I've been getting into cycling, as I really want to do a triathlon. I feel like you're not a true cyclist until a bunch of you can all sit together in your Lycra outside a cafe. I can only hope to get to that level one day. Cycling is still very new to me, and I'm still getting used to riding on the roads with cars around. When Art came with me on my first ride on the road, I cried twice within about 3 kilometres, because I was so nervous and wobbly around the cars. Now, I'm pleased to report, I can head off by myself quite happily, and I'm not such a crybaby.

PUT YOUR FEET UP

Allowing your body time to rest is just as vital as keeping active, because it gives your muscles time to repair and build (which can't be a bad thing). Rest is also just as important for your mind. If you go too hard every day, there's a high chance you will burn yourself out before too long. That's when you stop enjoying exercise and start to resent it—and that can leave you dangerously close to chucking in the towel and going back to old, unhealthy habits.

If you're not sure when to have a rest day, just listen to your body: it will let you know. If you're feeling tired and don't feel like doing any exercise, then don't! Take the day off. Give your body the time it needs to recharge its energy levels. I usually find that I feel much stronger and more energetic after a couple of days off, as though my body has fresh batteries.

You may have noticed I included pancakes on my Sunday workout schedule in the box on page 135. No, that wasn't a mistake. I *love* pancakes. I don't believe it's necessary to cut out every single food that you love—even if it's something that might traditionally be thought of as 'unhealthy'. If you cut yourself off from every food you love, you'll go crazy, and life would be boring! Pancakes make everything better! Use your treat foods as a reward for looking after yourself, and you will enjoy them even more.

EYES ON THE PRIZE

I find that setting fitness goals is a great way to keep myself motivated long term when it comes to exercise. I like to sign up for fitness events throughout the year—big or small—so that I always have something to work towards. As I mentioned, not that long ago I signed up for the Auckland half-marathon and I found it really beneficial to have that extra bit of motivation, knowing I had an event coming up, to help me stick with my running.

For my training, I started with three small runs a week of no more than 5 kilometres, then went for one big run on the weekend. Week by week, I slowly increased the distance of the long run until I was running about 16 kilometres just before the race.

(If you're thinking of giving a half-marathon a go yourself, you can find lots of free beginners' training programmes online.)

The week before the half-marathon event, Art and I went to Fiji for AccorHotels Fiji Race to Survive, a Cure Kids event that is sort of like a mix between *The Amazing Race* and *Survivor*. We had a week of physical exertion and minimal sleep, so I was slightly worried that I wouldn't have the energy for the half-marathon—but, as it turned out, that proved to be the least of my worries! In our last couple of days in Fiji, I managed to pick up a stomach bug, and let's just say I preferred to be near a toilet at all times. (Because I had explosive diarrhoea, in case you didn't pick that up.)

Anyway, we headed home and the morning of the half-marathon rolled around. I wasn't feeling much better, but I had worked so hard towards doing the race that *not* doing it just wasn't an option. As I stood at the start line, I felt that unmistakeable pain deep in the depths of my stomach and I knew that I needed to find a loo quick-smart. I went and stood in the 100-person-long public toilet queue, but when I finally got to the cubicles I discovered there were only two of them and the line behind me was still massive. I was far too embarrassed to do what I needed to do, so I held it in, and just went back and started the run.

All went well, for a while . . . until I felt

Witness the fitness

Following is an example of my weekly fitness routine. This is by no means what I do every week, nor is it even very strict—it's really more of an idea of what a week might look like for me (without distractions).

Monday: a spin class in the morning or at lunchtime if it's raining, or a cycle outside if it's nice weather.

Tuesday: one of my at-home workouts (see page 139–141) when I wake up.

Wednesday: a 30- or 40-minute run in the morning, and maybe a Pilates or functional-fitness gym class in the evening.

Thursday: rest.

Friday: spin class in the morning, or cycle outside if it's a nice day.

Saturday: run if it's sunny, otherwise an at-home workout.

Sunday: rest and pancakes.

that pang again. I was forced to make a detour into the home of a poor, unsuspecting family who had come outside to cheer people on. Little did they know when they headed out to the footpath that morning that they would have a stranger run in, poo in their house, then run out again! That happened twice. If you are the people who let me use your loo that day, I'm very sorry.

Anyway, possibly a little too much detail there . . . so let's get back to talking about exercise.

Even though the Auckland half-marathon was slightly traumatic, I still really enjoyed the day as a whole. There's such a buzz around sporting events, and everyone is so supportive of each other. It's a really cool vibe. The first sporting event I ever did was a 5 kilometre fun run in London that was raising money for breast-cancer research. I was quite nervous, as I was doing it by myself and I had never run 5 kilometres before, but by the time I got there I realised that no one was judging me. It wasn't scary at all! There were people standing all along the sidelines, cheering the runners on, and it was amazing to see people come out to support each other. I remember the feeling of crossing the finish line so clearly! That event in particular made me realise just how amazing sporting events are. It's important to remember that the spectators and other competitors are all there to support you, not judge you.

Nowadays I like to do events with other people, whether with Art or with my friends. It's more fun if you have a training partner or two. Art wants to do that triathlon with me, so as I write this we have (slowly) started training. You know what they say about couples who train together? They probably fight a lot. (Kidding! They stay together.) Doing an event with someone else makes it so much more fun. Depending on what event you choose to do, the training can be gruelling, so having someone to keep you company and to go through all the hard work with you is hugely beneficial, and it helps keep you motivated.

The great thing about fitness events is that there are so many out there that you can find one to suit pretty much any fitness level. There's everything from 100 kilometre ultra marathons for elite athletes to 5 kilometre fun runs held all throughout the country.

At the end of the day, the best exercise you can do is one that you enjoy. Find what is sustainable for you, and do that. You will start to have more energy, be more positive, feel less stressed and even sleep better. Make living an active lifestyle a priority and you won't look back!

In the following pages, you'll find a couple of my favourite workouts. You can do these at home, at the park or at the gym.

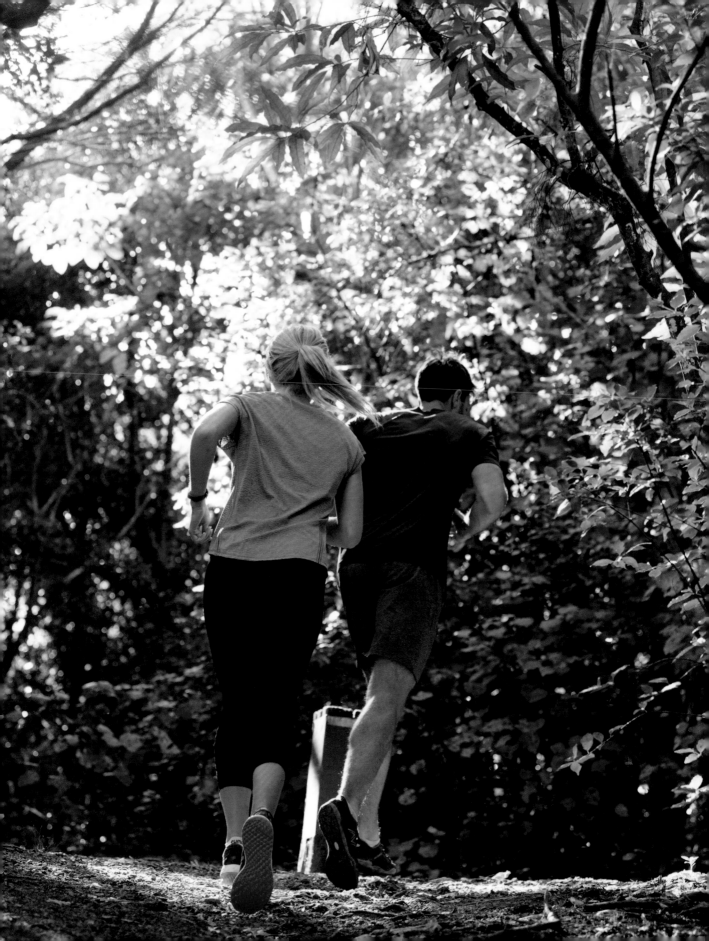

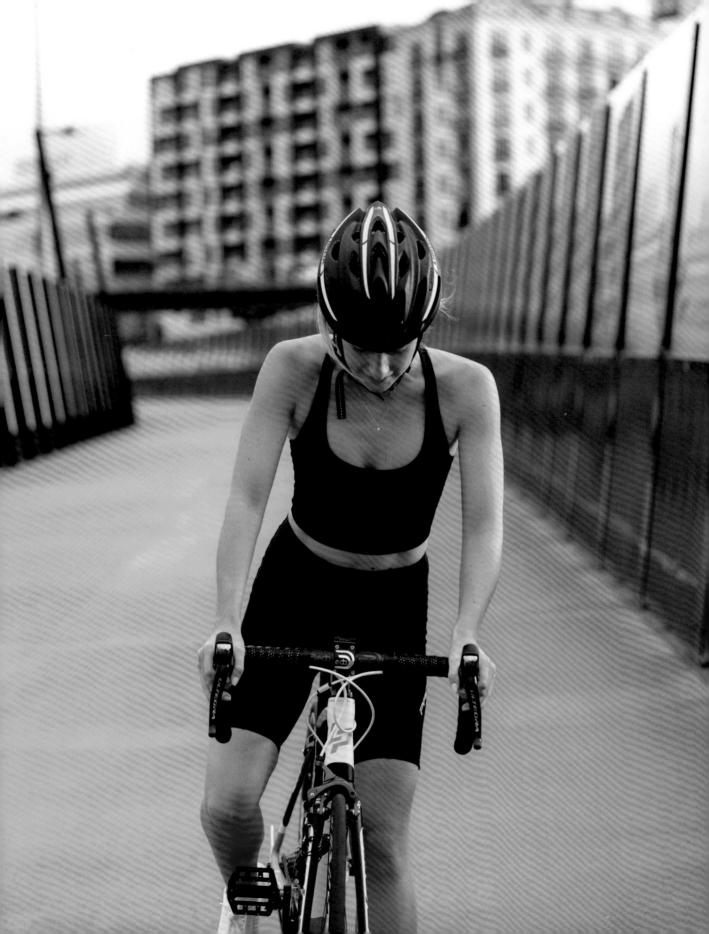

WORKOUTS

The following workouts are two of my favourites. They're especially great because you can do them anywhere and they don't take long at all. You can find detailed instructions for each of the exercises on pages 142–151.

These workouts use functional body-weight exercises—in my opinion, the most efficient way to train. It combines cardio and strength training, as well as burning fat quickly, and is also challenging for all fitness levels.

What I especially love about functional workouts is that you can get creative with them. These are workouts that I have put together (obviously), but once you've got the hang of the exercises you can mix and match and create your own workouts.

You can fit these workouts into your weekly exercise regime whenever you feel like mixing it up, or you can aim to do them around three times a week. It's totally up to you.

The ladder workout

This workout is super simple and any of the exercises can be substituted for any other exercise you prefer or feel like doing. It's a good idea to do two exercises that work different areas of your body, so that you're not just smashing your legs, or your arms.

Once you've done this one a few times, try going back through it in reverse and see how you go. (Spoiler alert: it's tough.)

- ♡ 10 x burpees and 1 x V sit-up
- ♡ 9 x burpees and 2 x V sit-ups
- ♡ 8 x burpees and 3 x V sit-ups
- ♡ 7 x burpees and 4 x V sit-ups
- ♡ 6 x burpees and 5 x V sit-ups
- ♡ 5 x burpees and 6 x V sit-ups
- ♡ 4 x burpees and 7 x V sit-ups
- ♡ 3 x burpees and 8 x V sit-ups
- ♡ 2 x burpees and 9 x V sit-ups
- ♡ 1 x burpee and 10 x V sit-ups

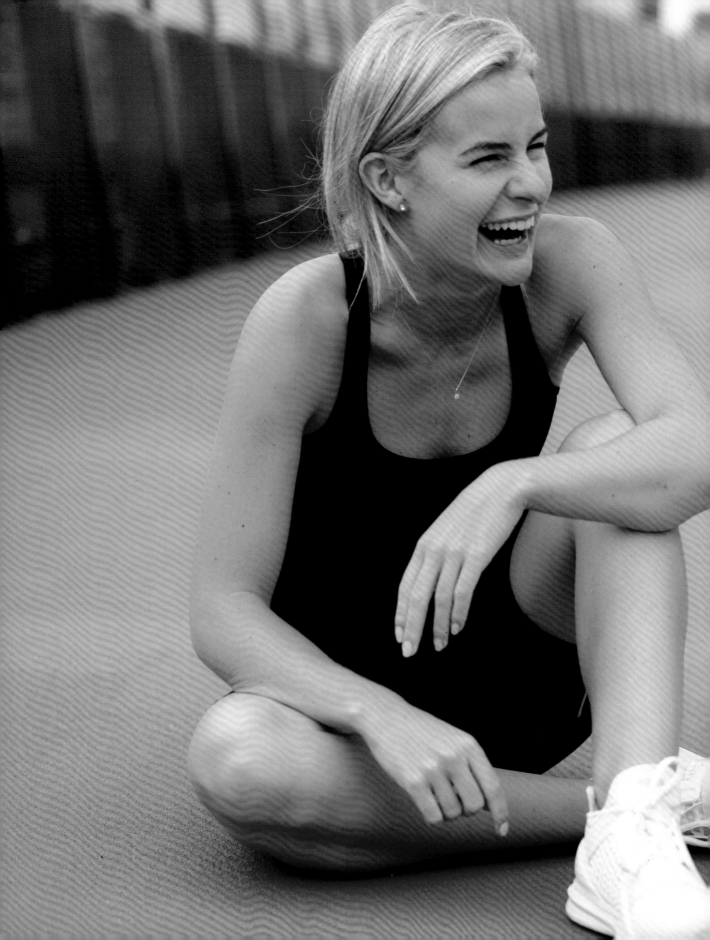

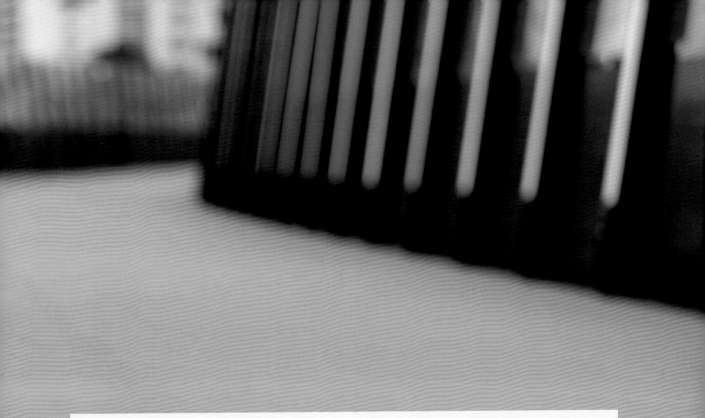

The fifteen-rep workout

A lot of these movements incorporate your whole body, and I've designed this workout to be short and sharp. It is high intensity and will get your heart rate up—and hopefully get a good sweat going too, because who doesn't love that? I prefer workouts like this one, which only use your body weight, as you can do them anywhere.

The whole thing should only take around ten or fifteen minutes.

If you're a beginner, just go through it once the first time, and work your way up to doing it twice. Then, once you're feeling fitter and stronger, hit it three times!

Enjoy!

- ♡ 15 x jump-squats
- ♡ 15 x push-ups
- ♡ 15 x starbursts
- ♡ 15 x burpees
- ♡ 15 x ice skaters
- ♡ 15 x bicycle abs
- ♡ 3 x bear crawls for 5 metres each
- ♡ 15 x sumo pulses
- ♡ 15 x split-jumps
- ♡ 15 x tricep push-ups
- ♡ 15 x supermans
- ♡ 15 x V sit-ups
- ♡ 15 x plank side-dips
- ♡ 1 x 60-second plank

THE EXERCISES

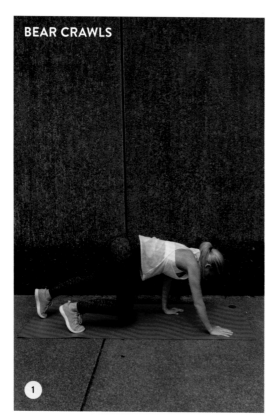

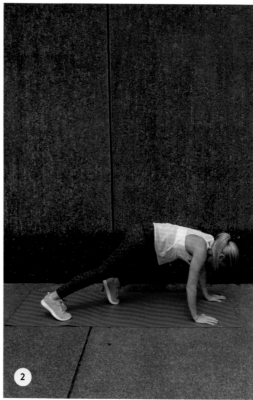

BEAR CRAWLS

Bear crawls

1. Start on all fours, with your hands straight out under your shoulders and your knees bent.
2. Walk along on all fours (like a bear), but don't let your knees touch the ground. Try to keep your bum down and your back as parallel to the ground as you can.
3. Do five lengths of about 5 metres each, backwards and forwards. (One 5 metre length equals one rep.)

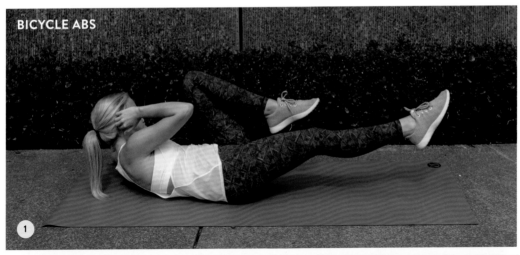

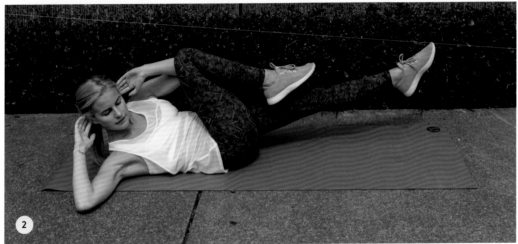

Bicycle abs

1. Lie flat on the floor, with your lower back pressed into the ground. (Pull in your belly button to target your deep abs as well.)
2. Put your hands behind your head, then bring your knees in towards your chest and lift your shoulder blades off the ground, but be sure not to pull on your neck.
3. Straighten your right leg out at a 45-degree angle to the ground, while turning your upper body to the left and bringing your right elbow towards the left knee. Make sure your rib cage is moving and not just your elbows!
4. Now do the same motion on the other side to complete one rep.

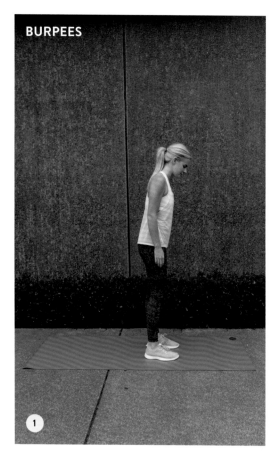

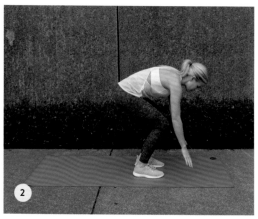

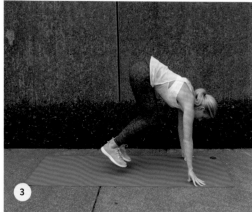

BURPEES

Burpees

1. Stand with your feet shoulder-width apart and your arms at your sides.
2. Push your hips back, bend your knees and lower your body into a squat (as though you were sitting down).
3. Place your hands on the ground directly in front of you and just inside your feet, and shift your weight onto your hands.
4. Jump your feet backwards to softly land on the balls of your feet in a plank position. Your body should form a straight line from your head to your heels. Now lower yourself down so your chest touches the ground, then push yourself back up again.
5. Jump your feet back in so that they land just outside of your hands.
6. Jump up explosively, reach your arms over your head and clap, to complete one rep.
7. Land in a squat position, ready to immediately start the next rep.

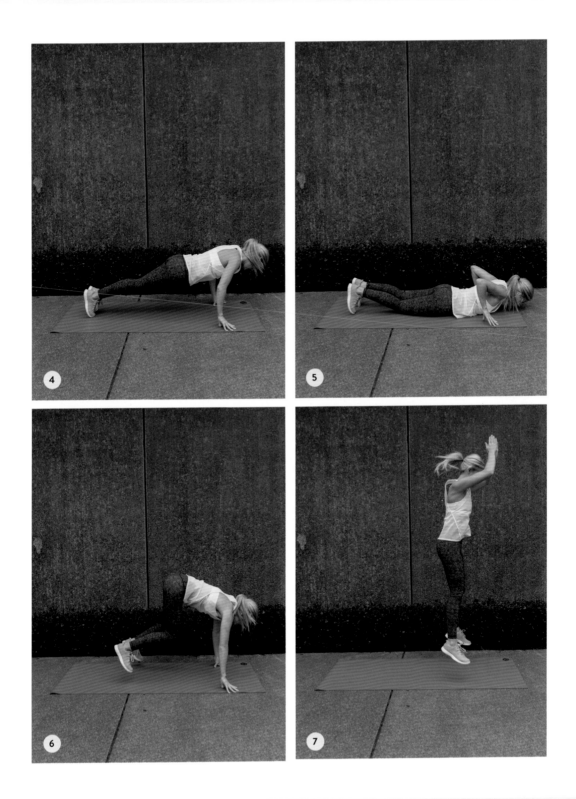

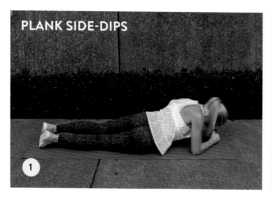 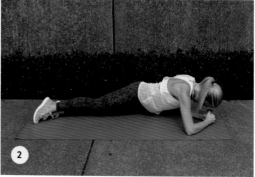

PLANK SIDE-DIPS

Plank side-dips

1. Get into a plank position on the ground, with your back as straight as you can and your elbows under your shoulders.
2. Slowly roll one hip to the side until it touches the ground. Make sure you are engaging your core and using your abdominals for this exercise, so you take the pressure off your lower back.
3. Use your abdominals to lift your hips back to a plank position to complete one rep, then repeat on the other side.

Ice skaters

1. Start standing on one leg.
2. Hop from side to side, switching legs as if you were hopping over a puddle or speed-skating. Swing your arms from side to side, the opposite arm going towards the opposite standing leg, and lowering your body down as you do so. (You've done one rep after you've hopped once on each foot.)

Jump-squats

1. Stand with your feet shoulder-width apart.
2. Start by doing a normal squat, then engage your core and jump up explosively.
3. When you land, lower your body back into the squat position to finish one rep. Land as quietly as you can—this requires control!

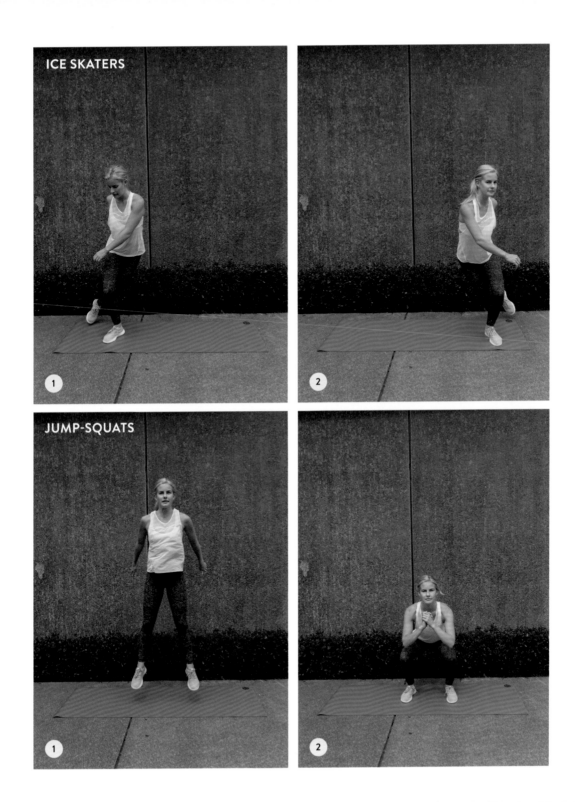

ICE SKATERS

JUMP-SQUATS

147

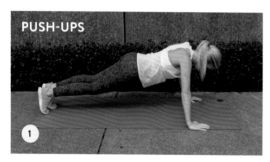 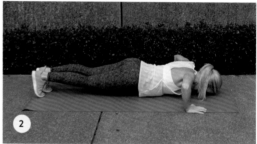

Push-ups

1. Get into a high plank position, with your hands firmly on the ground and directly under your shoulders.
2. Begin to lower your body, keeping your back flat and eyes focused about 8 centimetres in front of you to keep your neck neutral, until your chest just touches the floor.
3. Push back up to complete one rep.

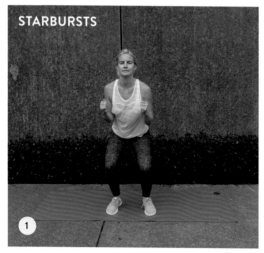 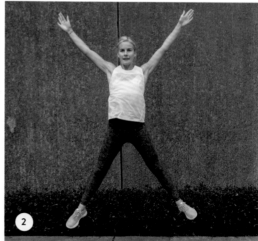

Starbursts

1. Stand tall, with your feet shoulder-width apart and your arms by your sides.
2. Bend down into a slight squat, then jump up explosively, raising your arms in the air and pushing both legs out to the sides.
3. As you land, bring both legs and arms back into a slight squat position to complete one rep. Again, try to land quietly to keep it controlled.

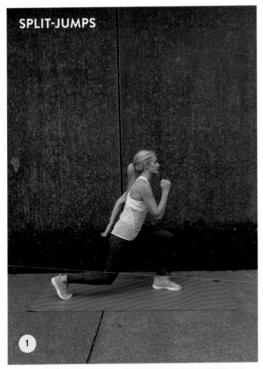

SPLIT-JUMPS

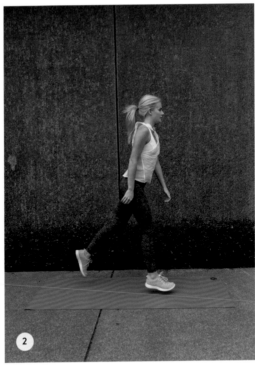

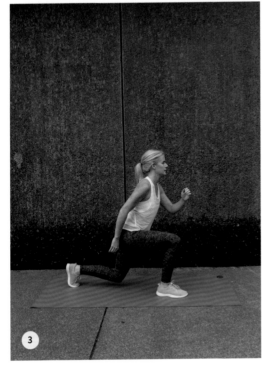

Split-jumps

1. Assume a lunge stance, with one foot forward and the knee bent, and the rear knee bent and nearly touching the ground. Ensure that your front knee is over the midline of your front foot and doesn't go over your toe.

2. Extending through both legs, jump as high as possible, swinging your arms to gain lift.

3. Switch legs in midair, then land softly on the other leg to complete one rep.

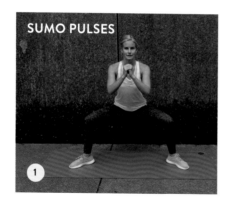

Sumo pulses

1. Start in a deep squat, with your legs opened wide out to the sides and your toes turned slightly outwards.
2. Holding that position, pulse a little up and down, moving only a couple of centimetres. Make sure not to let your knees go over your toes. (One pulse equals one rep.)

Supermans

1. Lie on the ground face down, with your arms stretched out in front of you.
2. Simultaneously raise your arms, legs and chest off the floor, and hold like this for two full seconds.
3. Slowly lower your arms, legs and chest back down to the floor to complete one rep.

Tricep push-ups

1. Get into a high plank position, and place your hands in a diamond shape on the floor in line with your shoulders.
2. Lower yourself until your chest almost touches the floor.
3. Using your triceps (the muscles at the back of your upper arms) and some of your pectoral muscles (the big muscles in your chest), press your upper body back up to your starting position, then squeeze your chest to complete one rep.

V sit-ups

1. Start by lying on your back, with your arms stretched above your head and your legs straight.
2. Using your abdominals, lift your legs, arms and torso at the same time into a V position. If you can touch your toes, do that, but it's not essential.
3. Keeping your abdominals engaged, slowly lower yourself back down to your starting position to complete one rep.

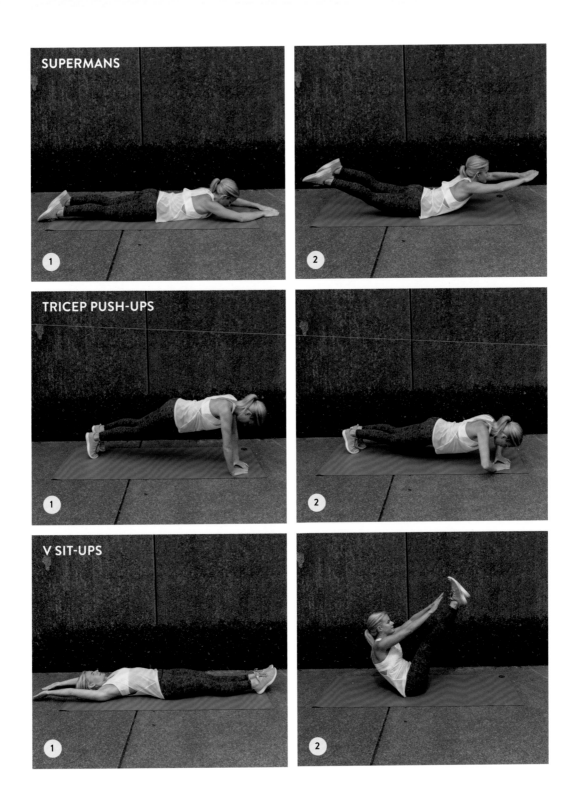

SUPERMANS

TRICEP PUSH-UPS

V SIT-UPS

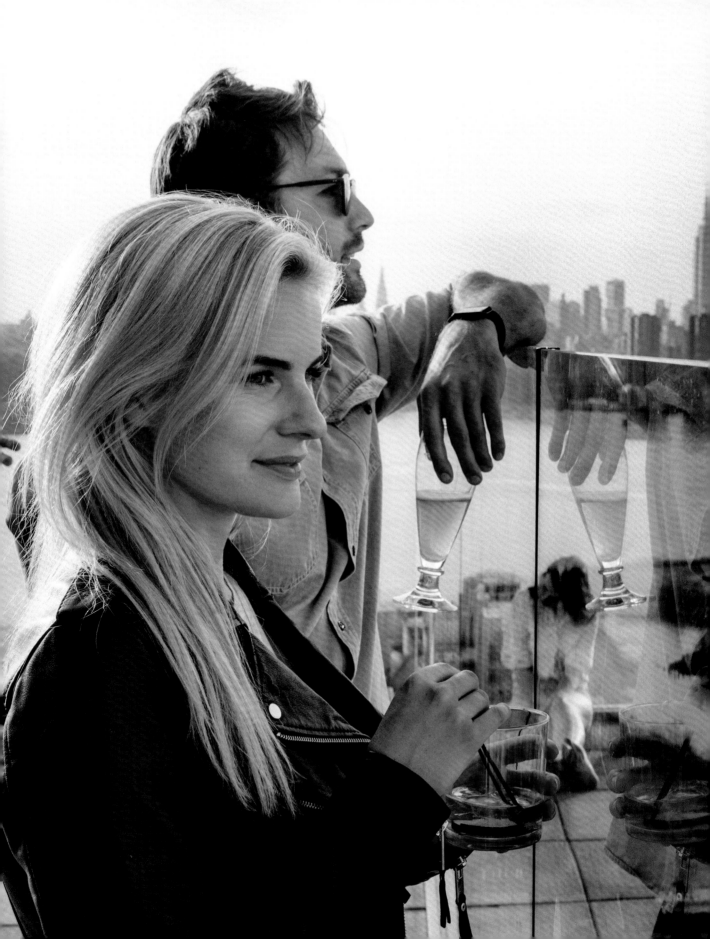

FINDING YOUR STYLE

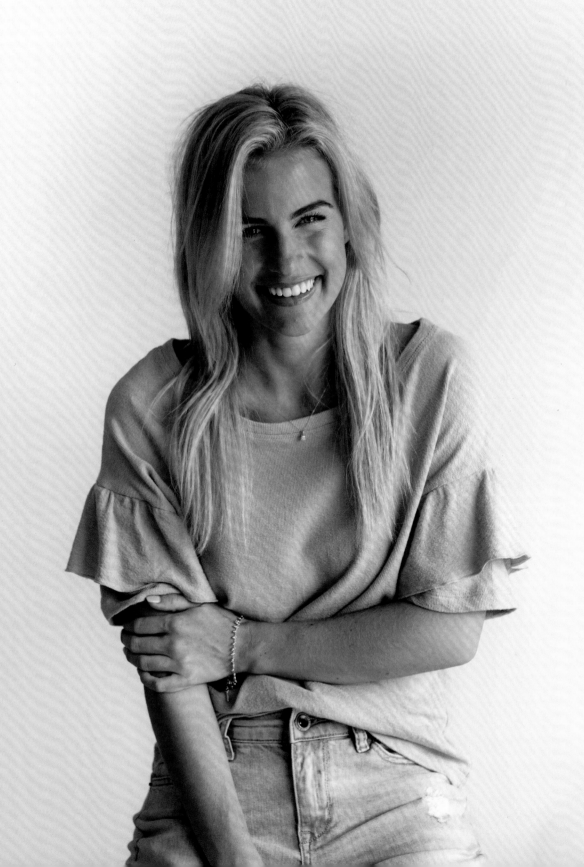

I have gone through so many different stages in my life when it comes to fashion and beauty. It can take a long time to figure out what your true style identity is, and I believe it's something that comes with age.

When I was a teenager, and even a little into my twenties, I was still figuring out what my own personal style was. I would mostly follow trends and copy what my friends were wearing, without really taking the time to get to know what colours suited me or what shapes were flattering (or not) for my body shape.

Now, I feel like I've finally reached a place where I have quite a distinct style. I would describe it as classic with a feminine touch, and I especially love light colours and simple designs. My friends always tease me for buying things that are a similar colour: pale pink, cream and grey marle in particular. I just love pastel colours, OK? So sue me!

HAVE SOME FUN WITH IT

I reckon that experimenting with and finding your own sense of style is one of the great joys of life. Figuring out your personal style is so important, as the impact goes far beyond just making a good first impression. Great style is also about approaching each day with confidence, and about being able to feel unstoppable in what you are wearing. The right wardrobe can increase your confidence in droves!

A good way to figure out your personal style is to pull everything out of your wardrobe that you *love*—maybe the top-ten outfits that you wear most often—and lay them on your bed.

Take a good, long look at the clothes in front of you. What trends can you spot? What similarities are there between them? And is there anything about them that's especially unique? Are there any colours or shades that pop up more than once? Are there any patterns, like stripes or polka dots? And what kinds of items are they—mostly dresses? Or jeans and sweaters? Or dress pants and shirts? Make a list of every trend and similarity you see, so you can further define them. That's your style.

Those outfits on your bed are obviously the outfits that you feel your best in, so keep them in mind when you're shopping for anything new. You can buy as many different and funky things as you like, but if you never wear them then they are not you. They're not your personal style. You might discover that you're really into getting glammed up when the occasion calls for it, or maybe you're a jeans and sweatshirt kind of person and feel happiest when you're in those comfy clothes. Whatever your thing is, go with it and embrace it. That's all part of finding your own style.

GETTING IT RIGHT

I don't think you can ever judge another person's outfit as 'wrong', because whether it's 'right' or not all comes down to how *they* feel in it. It doesn't really matter what anyone else thinks. Whenever I feel amazing in an outfit, that's when I know that I've got it right. You know that feeling when you're loving what you're wearing *and* you feel super confident about your ability to conquer whatever the day throws at you? Yep, that's the power of a good outfit, and that's how I measure whether I've got it right or wrong.

There have been countless times when I haven't been quite sure of an outfit . . . then, some time later, I'll look back and I can see why! Years ago, for instance, there was this trend for baby-doll boob-tube tops. (For those of you who aren't familiar with this particular item of clothing, it's a top that is tight around the bust and loose around the waist.) I looked like a box in them. They didn't suit me at all, and deep down I knew it, but I chose to ignore that and wore them anyway. Nowadays I know straight away that if I'm not sure of an item of clothing then I shouldn't wear it!

I had pretty terrible style during high school, actually. I remember in sewing class one year we had to make a top of some description. I chose to make a tight singlet that tied up at the back with a ribbon. I used this heinous pink metallic fabric that turned out to be really hard to sew, so the workmanship was quite shoddy. Plus I forgot to get a ribbon to tie it up at the back, so I used a shoelace instead. Yep, a shoelace.

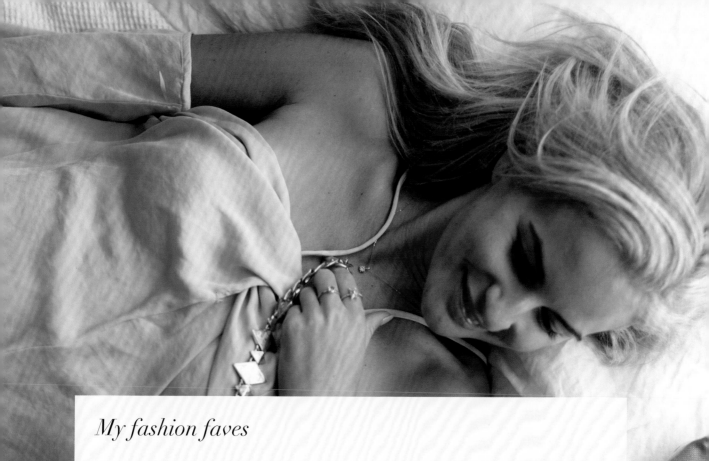

My fashion faves

♡ **A go-to pair of jeans.** My current personal favourite is a pair of boyfriend-style jeans, which are super comfortable and a really relaxed fit. I wear them during the day with a cool T-shirt or shirt and sneakers, but also dress them up with heels for an edgy night-time look. It doesn't matter what style your jeans are, so long as they fit you like a glove.

♡ **A white shirt.** I'm obsessed with shirts. I think they are so flattering on a woman! I have so many different shirts (not all white), as they are so versatile—you can wear a shirt to a board meeting, but also with denim shorts in summer.

♡ **A leather skirt.** Every girl needs a leather skirt. They are a staple that goes with everything, as well as looking super sleek.

♡ **A good hat.** A hat can take an ordinary outfit to the next level! I'll wear a hat to make a plain-ish outfit a bit more exciting, but hats are also great if you haven't washed your hair. You can get wool fedoras for winter, or straw hats for summer.

♡ **A classic pair of flats.** Whatever your style is, you need an everyday shoe that is comfortable, will never date and will go with everything.

Accessory tips

I know that accessorising can be hard if you're not used to adornments, and even pretty scary. So here are some of my personal 'rules', which I usually follow when I'm picking out just the right accessory. (Although don't forget it can also be fun to break the rules sometimes when it comes to fashion.)

- **Invest in well-made, good-quality accessories.** Since you use accessories so much, and if you get the right ones you can usually use them for more than just one season, it makes sense to get good ones.

- **Don't be too matchy-matchy.** I don't think it matters if you match a couple of accessories sometimes, but try not to go overboard or you can end up looking like you bought your outfit as a package deal, with not much of your own flair added.

- **Less is more.** You've probably heard the saying 'Remove one accessory before you leave the house'. I think it's spot on. Some people love to add *lots* of accessories, but I prefer to stick to one or two pieces. Each to their own, of course, but if you have too many accessories, it can look a bit full on.

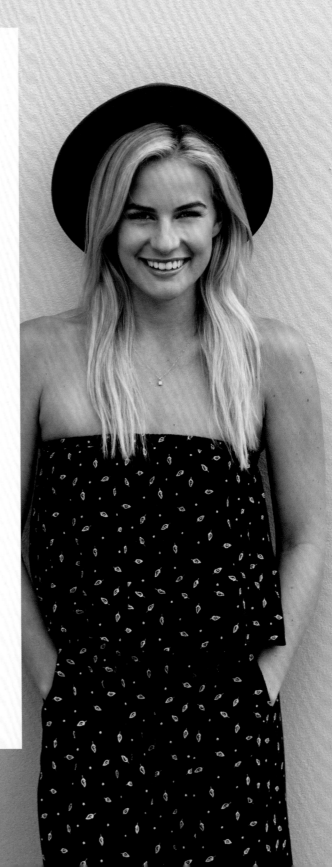

BORROWING ISN'T STEALING . . .

Like a lot of women, I'm bloody obsessed with Pinterest. I use it to get inspiration for everything: homewares, hair and make-up ideas and style. When it comes to fashion, I like to pay attention to what people whose style I admire are doing, then keep that in mind when I'm putting together my own outfits. I don't think there's anything wrong with getting inspiration from other people, as long as it's a style that you love, is personal to you and you aren't just blindly following what's 'cool' at the time.

I'm actually obsessed with English model and actress Rosie Huntington-Whiteley, as I think she has the most amazing style. Her outfit choices are always on point—she always looks so elegant, and never tacky. What especially stands out to me is how well she rocks denim and accessories.

Ah, denim. I love jeans, but I hate shopping for them. It's one of those less-enjoyable experiences of life, simply because it's so bloody hard to find the right pair! My main issue is usually that they are too loose around the waist but too tight around the thighs, or too tight around the waist but too loose around the legs. I know, first-world issues right here. I've learned that a good way to go when it comes to jeans is to find a brand that fits you perfectly, then use that as your go-to brand until the end of time. It's also worth spending the time trying on lots of different jean shapes, to figure out what looks best with your body shape. If they're on trend, but you don't feel good in them, don't wear them. In fact, that's just a good general rule of thumb when it comes to all things fashion.

DON'T BE AFRAID TO ACCESSORISE

I love a good accessory! The coolest thing about accessories is that the right ones can make you feel like your wardrobe has doubled in size. Since I like to dress quite simply, I find it fun to fluff up an outfit with some statement accessories, such as a really cool pair of sunglasses, some colourful shoes, a hat or an interesting scarf.

I have a collection of all of the above that I like to mix and match with all the time.

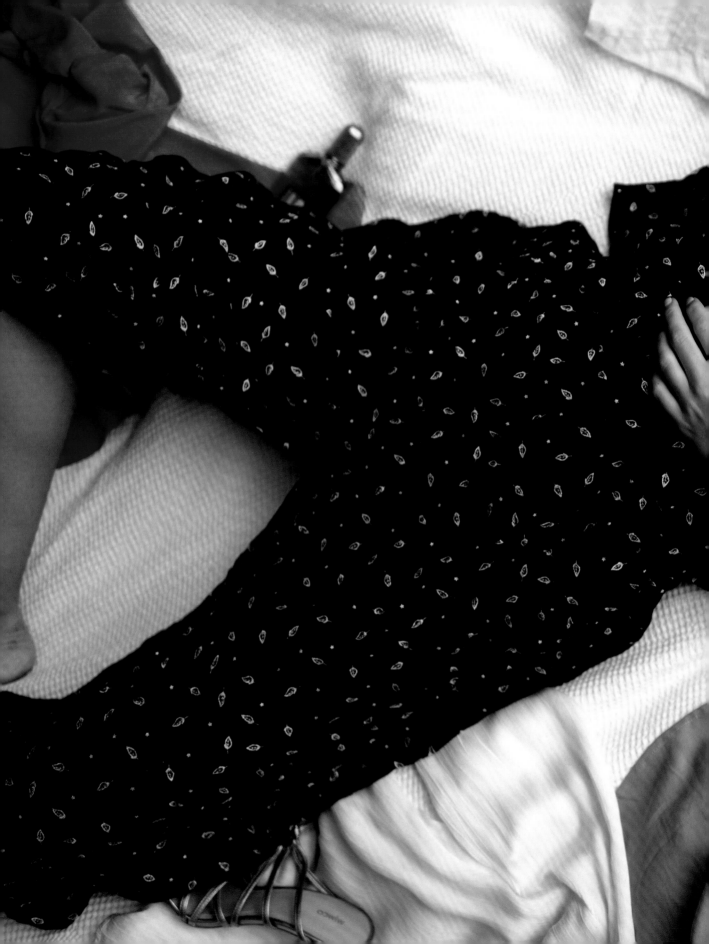

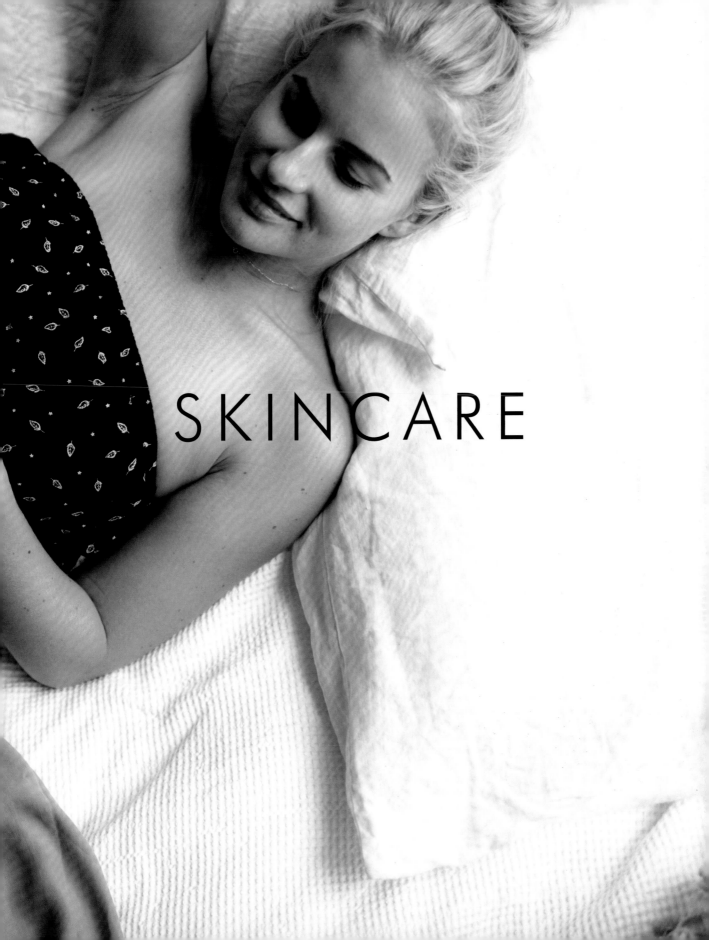

SKINCARE

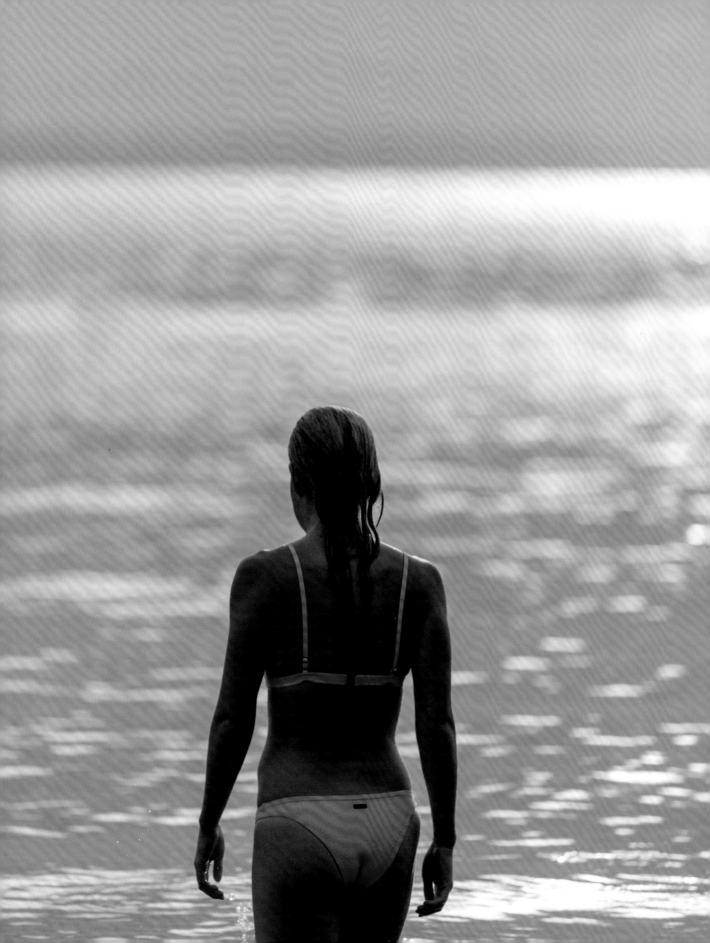

Bet you can't guess what the largest organ in your body is. I'll give you a moment to try to think of it . . .

Need a clue? It's right in front of your face. Well, on it, actually.

Still have no idea? OK, I'll stop prolonging this and just tell you: it's your skin! For real! (Also, the title of this chapter probably gave it away.)

The skin of an average-sized adult has a surface area of around 6.5 square metres, and it accounts for 6 to 10 per cent of your body weight. (Your second-largest organ, the liver, only accounts for about 2.5 per cent of your body weight.) As well as protecting your insides from outside nasties (and, importantly, keeping your insides where they are), your skin has a bunch of pretty crucial jobs:

- ♡ it helps regulate your body temperature
- ♡ it contains your nerve endings so that you can feel things
- ♡ it keeps you dry
- ♡ it stores lipids (fats) and water
- ♡ it absorbs oxygen, nitrogen and carbon dioxide (some animals even breathe entirely through their skin!).

When you bear all this in mind, it pretty much goes without saying that it is hugely important to look after your skin.

The skinny on skin

You might not have ever given your skin too much thought before, but you should. It's a pretty amazing thing!

- ♡ Each centimetre of your body contains around 8 million skin cells.
- ♡ Your body is constantly getting rid of dead skin cells and growing new ones—your body ditches about 35,000 skin cells every day!
- ♡ Hold up your hand. Take a good, long, hard look at the skin on it, cos it'll no longer exist in a month. It will have been *completely* replaced in that time.
- ♡ The top twenty or so layers of your skin are made up of dead cells, and the new ones form underneath this.

THE BASICS OF FACIAL SKINCARE

I believe that maintaining healthy skin is the key to looking radiant and feeling confident, so I take skincare *very* seriously. And it's important for everyone, not just the ladies—I've even got Art on to #skinregime2017. (He's on a strict regime of cleansing, toning and moisturising, with the odd exfoliation and, if I do say so myself, he is positively glowing.)

I think the basis of good facial skincare lies in being consistent with a routine, and there's no better time to start cementing a new habit than right now. Here are the top three things that I try to do in order to maintain healthy, glowing skin.

1. Drink LOTS of water—I'm talking 2 litres a day

I've found that doing this makes a *huge* improvement to my skin and my overall appearance. Keeping well hydrated is said to improve the elasticity of your skin, and I definitely find that it gives my skin that lovely 'plump', moisturised look and stops it from looking dry and dull.

2. Never, ever sleep in your make-up!

It's important to let your skin breathe overnight, and it can't do that if it's still caked with foundation. Sleeping in make-up can also clog your pores and lead to breakouts or eye irritations. Ew. It only takes a minute—wash it off.

3. Invest in good-quality skin care.

Do your research and choose products that add vitamins and minerals to your skin, and don't simply strip it of its natural oils. Make sure you're not just falling for good marketing or pretty packaging, and take some time to find out what the active ingredients are before you drop a cash bomb on skincare that isn't really doing you the favours it might promise. (I've included my skincare routine on page 167 so you can see which products I like to use.)

———

I BELIEVE THAT MAINTAINING
HEALTHY SKIN ON YOUR FACE IS
THE KEY TO LOOKING RADIANT
AND FEELING CONFIDENT, SO I
TAKE SKINCARE *VERY* SERIOUSLY.

———

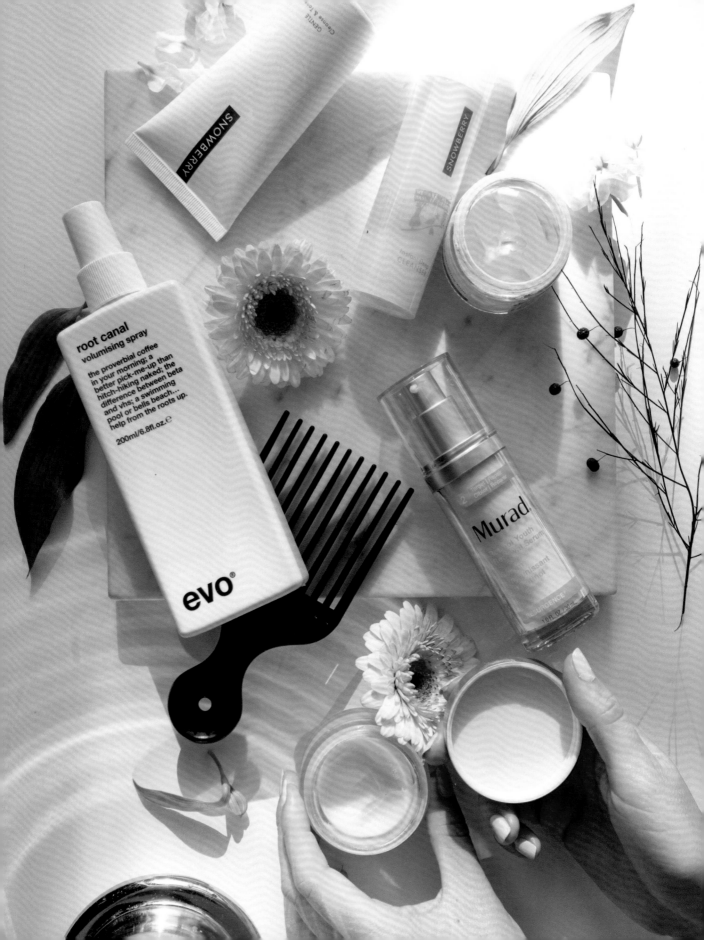

root canal
volumising spray

the proverbial coffee
in your morning; a
better pick-me-up than
hitch-hiking naked; the
difference between beta
and vhs; a swimming
pool or bells beach...
help from the roots up.

200ml/6.8fl.oz.℮

evo®

SNOWBERRY

Murad

My skincare routine

Every morning, I wash my face with **Snowberry Gentle Cleanser**, and I follow this with **Murad Hydrating Toner**. I like to use a gentle cleanser in the morning, as I don't need it to remove any make-up. I then put a tiny bit of **Murad Renewing Eye Cream** on my fingertip and dab it under my eyes and along my eyebrow line, which helps to reduce bags and dark circles under the eyes, and generally makes me look like I'm awake! Following that, I press some **Murad Retinol Youth Serum** onto my face, which firms the skin and helps to even out skin tone. Finally, I press in a tiny bit of **Tahi mānuka essential oil** as a natural moisturiser. Mānuka honey is a

great anti-inflammatory, reduces redness and also oxygenates pores to draw out bacteria, drastically improving acne-prone areas. Basically, it's a wonder product! If I'm not going to wear any make-up (all of my make-up contains an SPF), then I wear a light **Snowberry Everyday SPF 15 sunscreen** on my face.

At night, I sub out the gentle cleanser for **Snowberry Instant Deep Cleanser**, as it is a little more thorough at removing make-up and any dirt from the day, but otherwise my skincare routine is exactly the same as in the morning (without the sunscreen or make-up, obviously).

DON'T FORGET ABOUT
THE REST OF YOUR SKIN!

It's not that uncommon for people to pay close attention to caring for the skin on their face, but they often forget that the skin on their body needs love too!

I moisturise my body every day after my shower with a natural moisturiser, and during summer I make sure to use my Snowberry SPF 15 sunscreen every day (SPF 30 if I'm heading to the beach). I make sure to exfoliate my body every week or two in winter, and slightly less frequently in summer when I want to keep my tan. I don't like using anything on my body that's too heavily fragranced—no real reason; I just don't really like it!—so I prefer to make my own exfoliator, and I've given you my Full-Body Exfoliant recipe on page 169 if you want to give it a try yourself.

You can use it on your whole body, but if you do just make sure to apply it in the shower or bath, as it can be a little bit messy. Otherwise, I like to use it as a hand treatment: to do this, just massage it into your palms and hands while you are watching TV for at least five minutes (longer if you like), then wash it off. Your hands will feel incredible! I wouldn't recommend using this one on your face though, as it is probably a little harsh for your sensitive wee facial skin.

The quantities I've given might need adjusting, depending on how much of your body you are exfoliating—the best thing to do is to judge it for yourself and add more of each ingredient as you see fit, keeping the proportions the same. My recipe makes enough for your hands and maybe one other part of your body, like your legs or arms.

Press it in

I read somewhere years ago that you should never rub moisturisers or serums onto your face; instead, you should warm it in your hands first, then press it into the skin. I've since learned that gentle pressure in certain places on your face can also help creams, serums and oils be absorbed, and also stimulates lymphatic circulation, which clears toxins faster.

This is because you have these things called 'facial lymph nodes', which are like the ones in your armpits, but in your face. When you press with reasonable pressure in areas on your face, it helps these lymph nodes flush toxins from your body, helps drain sinuses, reduces fluid retention in your face, and can even help alleviate cold symptoms!

Not all areas of skin are created equal, though, and certain areas need to be given extra-special attention. I prefer to press product over my whole face, but if you want to you can also treat these specific areas with gentle pressure in a circular motion. The super-delicate skin around your eyes should never be rubbed, as that can cause the skin to darken and swell, leading to under-eye shadows and bagging; instead, gently pat your products into this area.

The areas to gently press are:
- under your jaw and down your neck to where your collarbones meet
- around your ears and sides of your nose; this movement helps to clear your sinuses
- starting at the inner corner of your eyebrow, gently press along under your eyebrow, and finish on the outer corner of your brow.

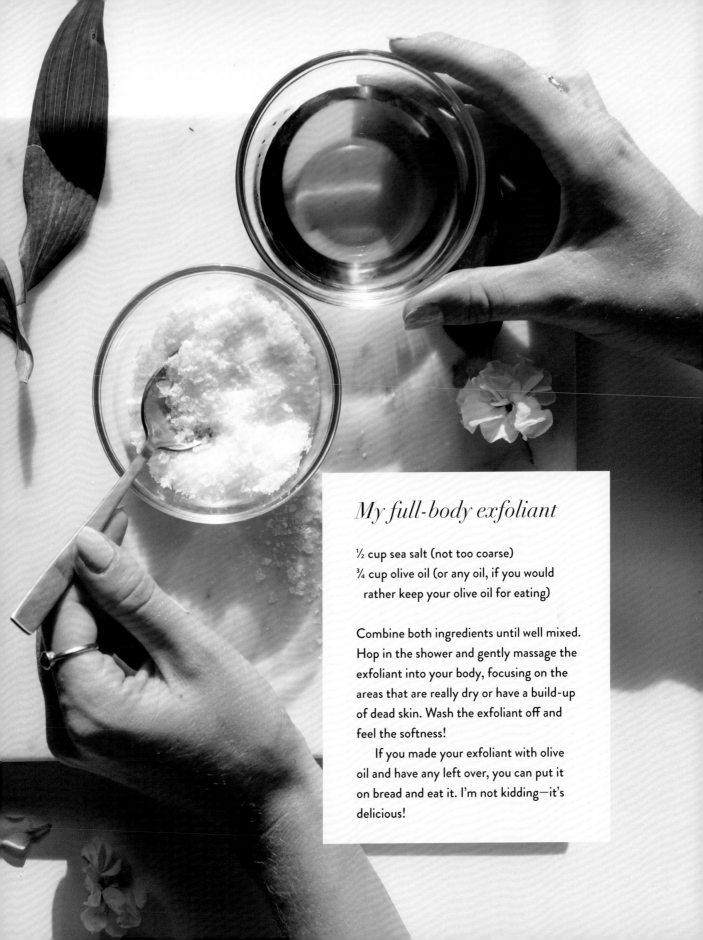

My full-body exfoliant

½ cup sea salt (not too coarse)
¾ cup olive oil (or any oil, if you would
   rather keep your olive oil for eating)

Combine both ingredients until well mixed.
Hop in the shower and gently massage the
exfoliant into your body, focusing on the
areas that are really dry or have a build-up
of dead skin. Wash the exfoliant off and
feel the softness!

   If you made your exfoliant with olive
oil and have any left over, you can put it
on bread and eat it. I'm not kidding—it's
delicious!

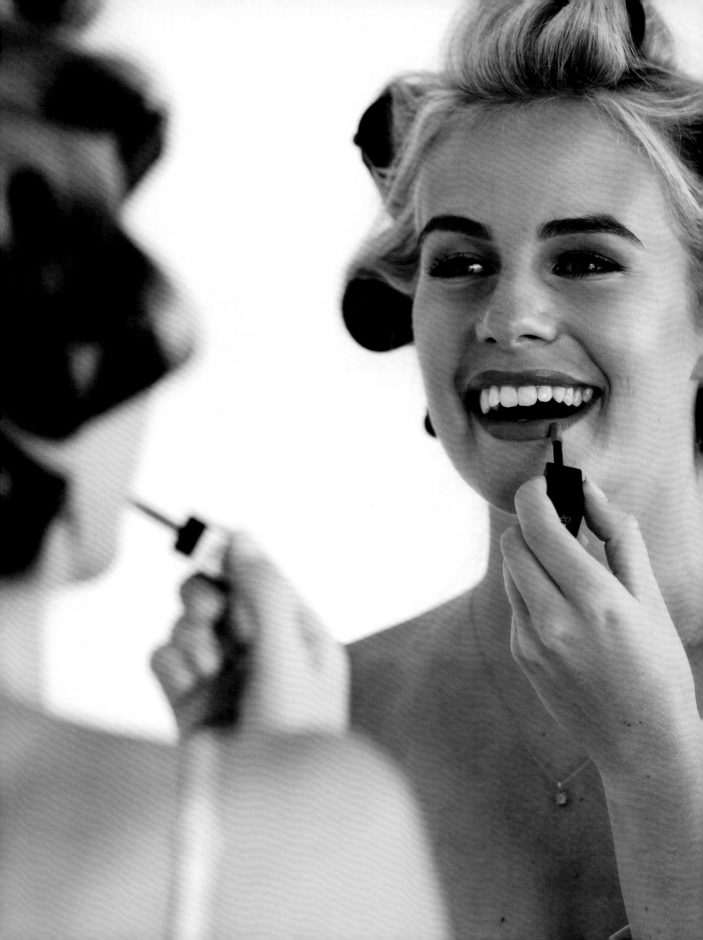

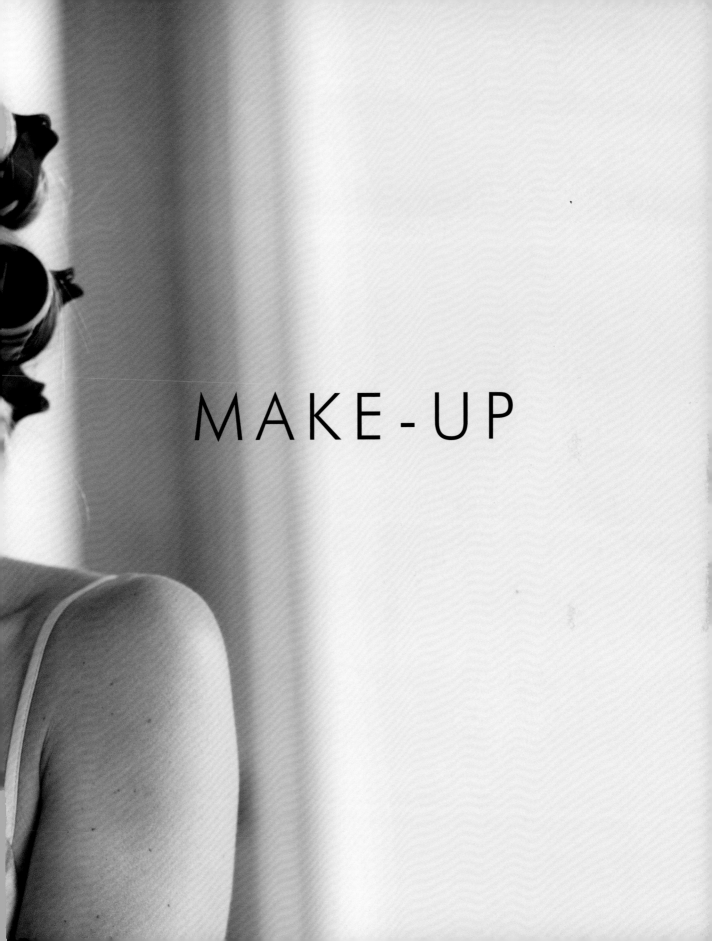

MAKE-UP

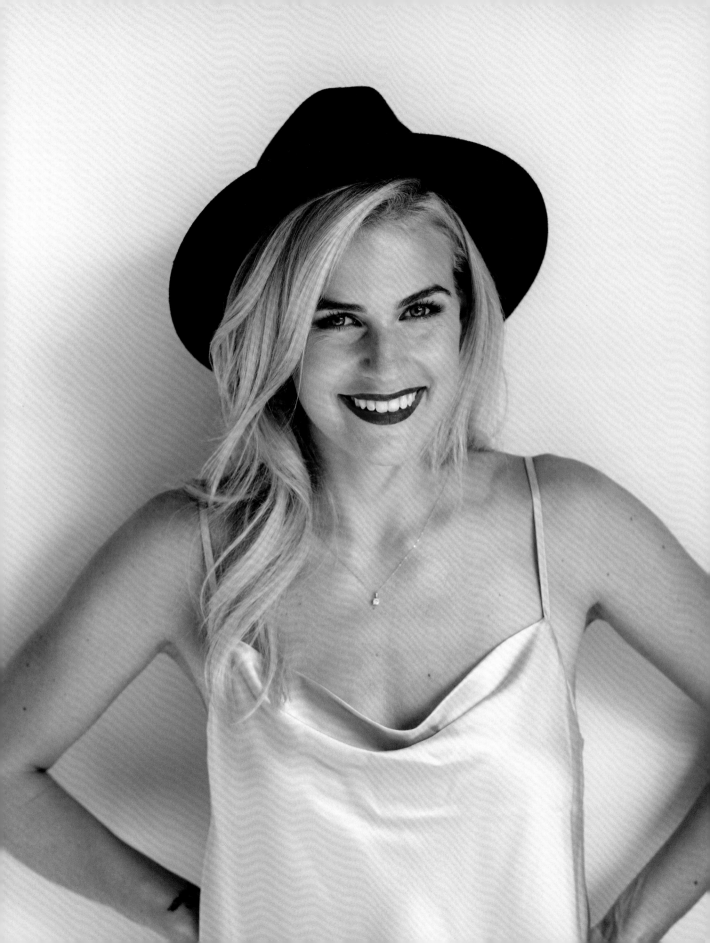

Make-up is fun! It's fun experimenting with different looks but, just like your wardrobe, it can sometimes take a little while to work out what your personal make-up style is— and, if you're anything like me, you might've had a few slightly embarrassing phases on your way to working out your style (I feel like you're not a human if you haven't). These days, I love getting glammed up if I'm going out in the evening or to a special event, but otherwise I tend to keep my make-up pretty low-key and natural. But that hasn't always been the case . . .

THE FAKE-TAN YEARS

I first started getting into make-up when I was about fourteen. When I say 'getting into make-up' what I really mean is 'getting into *Mum's* make-up': I would go through her cosmetic bag and use all of her products when she wasn't looking. Her foundation was about ten shades too dark for me as she is naturally far more tanned than I am, but I would wear it anyway. I believed it made me look 'tanned' too. (I'm yet to meet anyone who has a face that tans ten shades darker than the rest of their body.)

That was just the beginning. From that point on, my teenage years were filled with some massive make-up fails. I plucked my eyebrows into thin, straight lines across my face. I opted for the 'patchy and orange and far-too-much' make-up look. And then the stage started that I would really like to forget: the fake-tan stage.

When I tell people I was addicted to fake tan in my teenage years, they all say, 'Oh, me too! I went through that stage!'

Then I show them pictures, and their eyes widen and they are lost for words.

It all began when I was about seventeen. What can I say? I just got really obsessed with fake-tanning. I thought I looked *great*. It reached the point where I was parting with a stupid amount of money so I could spend half an hour a week spraying myself with fake tan in my room. My sheets were constantly soiled with fake tan and there seemed to be a thin layer of it over every inch of my bedroom and bathroom.

I'm sure my mum remembers that time fondly.

One day at work, I found some of my colleagues waiting for me.

'Matilda,' one of the ladies said kindly. 'We think it's time we had a chat.'

They wanted to talk about my tanning. They were staging a fake-tan intervention! It was *that* bad. People were so concerned about my fake-tan use that they felt the need to step in.

But I was in the full throes of fake-tan addiction, so I didn't listen to them. I didn't believe them. I thought I looked all kinds of fabulous, and I carried right on.

Then I went to my cousin's wedding. By this time, I was nineteen. Yep, I was two years deep in my fake-tan affair. I went off to the wedding in a nice dress, with my skin the usual shade of fake-tanned mahogany, and a face full of make-up that was about two inches thick. I felt great. I looked great (or so I thought).

A few weeks later, my cousin shared the official photos.

Oh, they're so nice! I was thinking as I admired the group shots. *Everyone looked so good. Wait—what's that?*

A brown smudge had caught my eye.

Is that . . . ?

I squinted a bit closer at the photo, then sat back with a gasp of alarm.

Lo and behold, that brown smudge was *me*!

That was the moment reality hit. At long last, it all became startlingly, shockingly clear: I had spent the last two years of my life looking absolutely ridiculous.

That very day, I started to cut back on the fake tan, and I also toned down the make-up situation.

These days, I still use fake tan from time to time—but I make sure to only use a tiny bit, to only apply one layer, and to go for a shade that isn't orange. I'm careful to make sure I don't relapse!

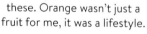

I actually have no words for these. Orange wasn't just a fruit for me, it was a lifestyle.

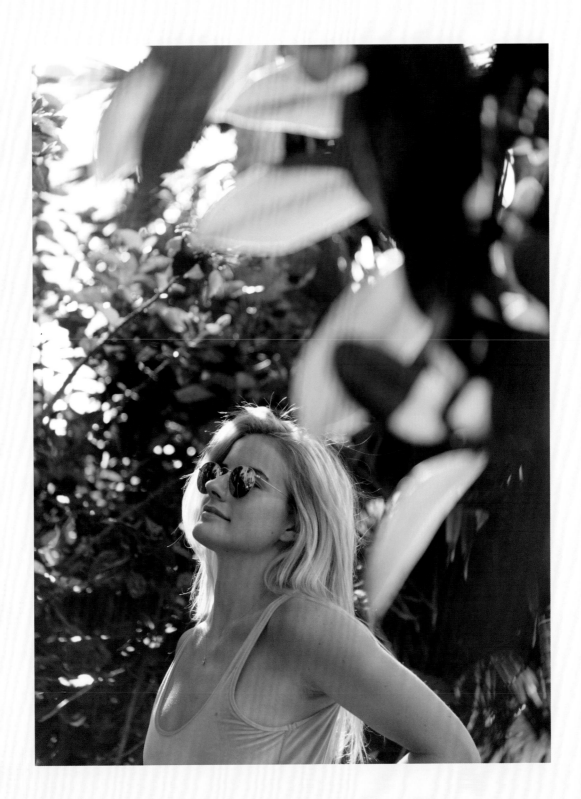

IT'S SO EMPOWERING WHEN
YOU REALISE THAT YOU NO
LONGER CARE WHAT OTHER
PEOPLE THINK, AND INSTEAD
FEEL CONFIDENT ENOUGH TO
DO WHAT FEELS NATURAL AND
RIGHT FOR YOU.

LESS IS MORE

I love nothing more than doing something special with my make-up for a night out, but during the day I prefer to wear no make-up at all as much as possible. Nowadays, I'm really happy to say that I am more comfortable in my own skin than ever before. I don't feel like I need make-up in order to be confident. The bonus is that it means my skin can breathe during the day. Plus I get ready *much* faster in the morning—which means more time in bed, and anything that results in more time in bed can't be a bad thing.

I got to a stage in my life a couple of years ago when I started to envy girls who wore no make-up. Up until that point, I'd always worn make-up every day, but then I just started to get sick of it! I realised that I didn't want to rely on wearing make-up, and I thought that getting rid of it might give me a confidence boost and help me to feel more comfortable in my own skin. So I gave it a shot.

When I first started going without any make-up during the day, I'd sometimes have people say unhelpful things to me like, 'You're looking a little pale', or 'You look a bit tired'. I found it quite hard to stick to my decision not to wear make-up after comments like that, and I'd be tempted to start wearing it again just to make the comments stop. However, I stuck with it, and over time I actually found that my skin slowly began to improve. As it did, I felt less and less like I needed to wear make-up. Eventually, I began to feel beautiful without make-up, and—best of all—I stopped caring what anyone else thought.

It's so empowering when you realise that you no longer care what other people think, and instead feel confident enough to do what feels natural and right for you. It takes time, but it's a cool and important place to get to. At the end of the day, it doesn't matter what anyone else thinks you do or don't look like; all that matters is that *you* feel good and happy in your own skin.

LIKE DAY AND NIGHT

I'm not saying I never, ever wear make-up during the day any more. It's not a hard-and-fast rule; it's just something I try to do most of the time. Sometimes I wake up in the morning and I feel like putting make-up on, so I do. If I have a dressy daytime event to go to, I will wear a little make-up for sure.

When I do opt for make-up during the day, I prefer to keep it light, as I think it's nice when someone's natural beauty still comes through. Make-up is not there to hide things; it's there to help what is already beautiful about you stand out. We (especially us ladies) seem to be programmed to pick out the things that we don't like about ourselves, but it's much more powerful and helpful to our overall well-being to focus on the things that we *do* like. Perhaps you really love your long eyelashes, so you'll use some good mascara to make them pop? Or maybe your cheekbones are your main asset, so you'll apply some light blush to bring them out? Whatever it might be that you think is already beautiful about yourself, use your make-up to show it off—not to cover up what you feel you don't like. You can find step-by-step instructions for how I achieve my all-time favourite daytime make-up look on page 183–186.

When I'm doing a night-time make-up look, I like to get a bit more creative. I don't hit the town all that often (I can be a bit of a nana), but when I do I love to wear a dark lipstick. There's just something so elegant and sexy about a striking lipstick! I especially love colours like plum, deep red and mahogany. I've shown you how I create my perfect evening look simply by adding to a natural daytime look on page 187–188.

My beauty product faves

I can be a bit of a beauty-product hoarder. I *love* beauty products and have so many at home. Admittedly, often I get drawn in by pretty packaging, but I mostly like products that have been recommended to me by a trusted source or are my kind of colour. Environmentally friendly brands are a huge bonus.

These are just some of my faves:

- **Inika foundation and bronzer.** Inika is a cruelty-free, organic brand of make-up, and this foundation is the best I've used. It's smooth and it leaves me with a lovely glow.
- **Maybelline Color Sensational Shaping Lip Liner** in Nude Whisper.
- **Nyx Butter Gloss** in Éclair.
- **Nyx Born to Glow Liquid Illuminator.** I love a good highlighter! I think it makes your skin look so fresh and dewy, and really brings out your cheekbones.
- **evo Root Canal Volumising Spray.** I was unfortunately born with naturally flat hair (I'm sure a lot of you are in the same boat), so I need to use product to puff it up a bit. This works really well. Just spray it into your roots before you blowdry, and voila! Instant volume.

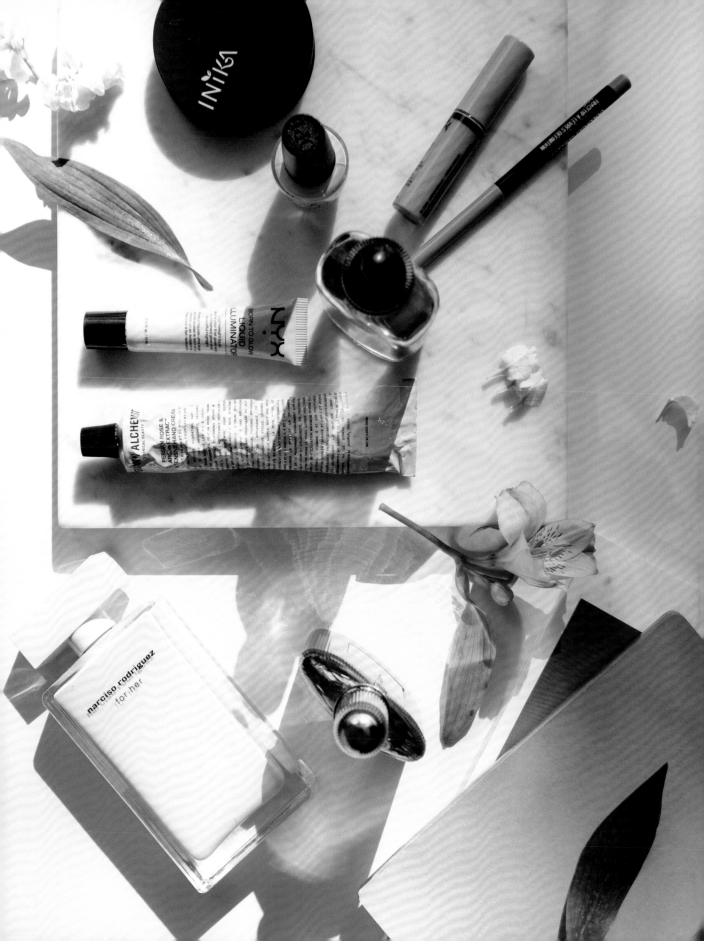

Nail your evening look

These are my tips for achieving the perfect evening make-up look that requires the least amount of effort for maximum effect!

♡ **Don't overdo the foundation.** Keep it at a light coverage, and make sure to use a primer foundation that achieves the look you want so you don't need a powder. A primer is a moisturiser designed to go underneath your foundation to help it stay on and look smooth and flawless. For example, if, like me, you prefer a dewy look, then use an illuminating primer; alternatively, if you prefer a matte look, then choose an oil-free mattifying primer. I'm not a fan of powder as it gets stuck in the creases in your face and can make you look older than you are. It also tends to flatten your features.

♡ **Go for *either* a statement lip colour *or* a statement eyeshadow or blush—never both.** It can be quite frightening if there's too much happening on your face. (There's also the potential to look a bit clown-like.)

♡ **Two words: lip liner.** Kylie Jenner showed me the benefits of lip liner and now I will never go back! If you don't follow her on Snapchat, you should; she's hilarious. And I've never seen such a lip transformation! (I suspect she may have had some help in the surgical department, but she still does wonders with a lip liner. Google it.)

♡ **Instead of eyeliner, apply a little of your eyeshadow along your bottom lash line.** This stops things looking too dramatic, but still brings out your eye colour.

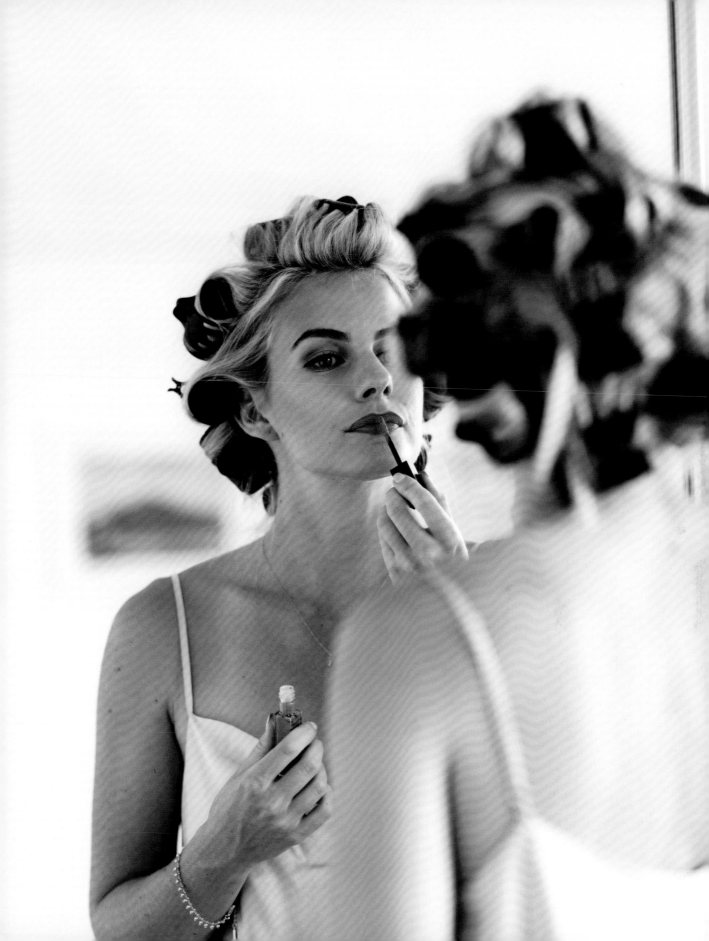

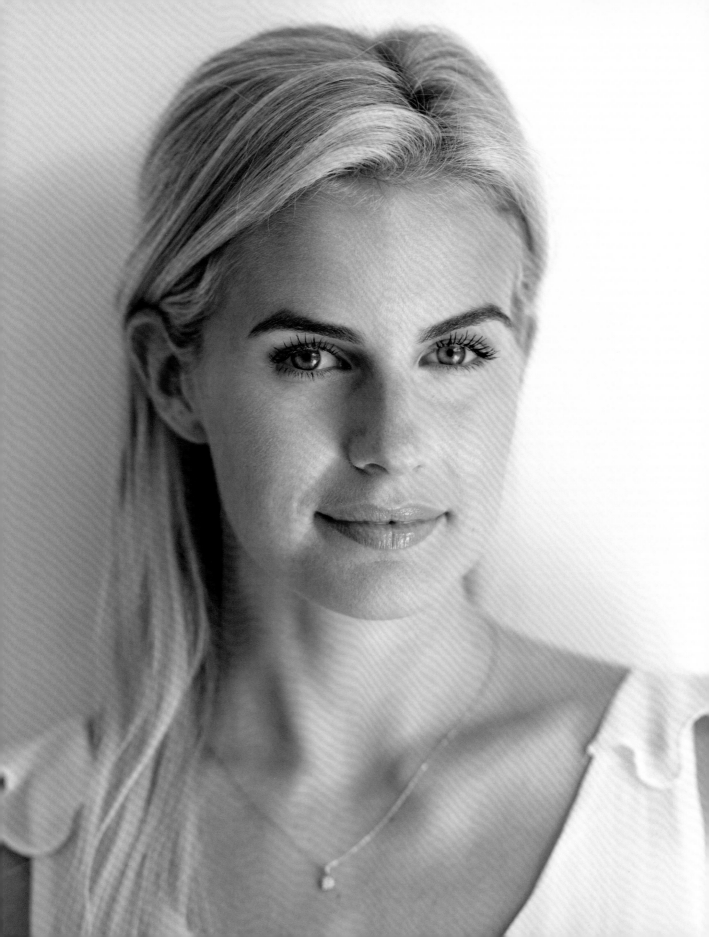

MAKE-UP
STEP-BY-STEPS

———

Here, I've outlined the steps involved in creating my go-to daytime and night-time make-up looks. Obviously, these are looks that I've developed because they go with my personal style and my colouring, but hopefully you can use them as inspiration to get your make-up out and start playing around to adapt your own go-to looks. Nothing beats sitting down in front of the mirror and giving things a go in the safety of your own bedroom or bathroom; there'll be some things that don't work, but if you give yourself time to experiment you'll also find the things that do work! Pinterest is my guilty pleasure for all things beauty. I could waste hours on that bloody app! I recommend scrolling through Pinterest and having a look at what other people who have your colouring are doing, and getting inspiration from them.

MY ALL-TIME FAVOURITE
DAYTIME LOOK

———

Daytime make-up is very different from an evening look. Make-up during the day needs to be much lighter. Daylight can make heavy make-up really obvious, and things can quickly look a bit scary. I'm a big believer in accentuating your features rather than covering up your face, so I prefer a lighter foundation coverage—and sometimes even just tinted moisturiser if I'm going for that no make-up look but don't feel like going totally make-up free. (Refer to the photo on page 182 if you need to for this look.)

Step 1:

MAKE SURE YOUR SKIN IS NICE AND CLEAN.

Before you do anything else, cleanse, tone and apply whatever moisturiser is going to work with the look you're trying to achieve. (See page 167 for my daily skincare routine.) I like to put a tiny bit of face oil on under my make-up, as I prefer a dewy, glowing look; if you prefer more of a matte look, then use an oil-free moisturiser.

Step 2:

APPLY YOUR FOUNDATION.

Here, I used **Inika Certified Organic Liquid Foundation**. You can apply your foundation with a brush or your fingers, but *please* make sure to blend it into your neck! Mainly to keep me happy, as foundation that's not properly blended is probably among my top-ten most hated things.

Step 3:

APPLY A LIGHTER CONCEALER UNDERNEATH AND TO THE INNER CORNERS OF YOUR EYES.

Here, I used **Maybelline Dream Lumi Touch Highlighting Concealer**, as it is light reflecting, which is great if you're feeling a bit tired and carrying a bit of extra baggage under those eyes. Applying concealer here will make you look much more awake.

Step 4:

APPLY A SMALL AMOUNT OF BRONZER TO YOUR TEMPLES, AND A TINY BIT JUST UNDER YOUR CHEEKBONES.

This frames your face, and also gives you a nice, healthy glow. Here, I used **Bobbi Brown Bronzer** in Golden Light.

Step 5:

TIME FOR EYESHADOW!

Using whichever eyeshadow palette you prefer (I like pink and purple shades for a daytime look), apply a layer of one of the lighter shades all over your eyelid. To add depth, take a slightly darker colour and apply it just along the crease of your eyelid. I like to shade this in a little more on the outer corner of my eyelid so that it gets lighter as it gets closer to the inner corner. Apply a thin layer of the darker eyeshadow along your bottom lash line to make your eyes stand out.

Step 6:

MASCARA TIME!

Apply mascara to your lashes. I'm sometimes guilty of putting too much on, so it starts to clump. Try to steer clear of that! Less is definitely more when it comes to mascara. In terms of which mascara you use, it's totally a matter of preference. Here, I've used **Maybelline The Colossal Big Shot** mascara, as it does amazing things for your lashes but also washes off easily. (I hate waterproof mascara, as it can seem to stay on like concrete.)

Step 7:

GET SOME BLUSH ON THOSE CHEEKS.

Every girl needs a bit of blush in her life. I feel like so many people think blush is only for middle-aged ladies, but they couldn't be more wrong! Just a tiny dusting on the apple of your cheeks is all you need. Here, I used **MAC Mineralize Blush** in Dainty.

Step 8:

FILL IN YOUR BROWS.

This is definitely optional, as some people don't need it, but those of us who have been growing our brows out since that 'skinny brows are in' stage a few years back need all the help we can get. Here, I used **Bobbi Brown Perfectly Defined Long-wear Brow Pencil** and filled in only the bald patches. It's important not to go overboard when filling in your brows—you want them to look natural, not like a cartoon character.

Step 9:

APPLY COLOUR TO YOUR LIPS.

For daytime, I would only ever go for a light pink or nude, as I think it is the most natural and classic for my colouring (but maybe you're braver than me). Here, I used **Maybelline Color Sensational Shaping Lip Liner** in Nude Whisper to outline my lips, then filled them in with **NYX Butter Gloss** in Crème Brulee.

And, just like that, you're done and ready to conquer the day!

MY PERFECTLY EASY
EVENING LOOK

This look is the ultimate lazy girl's life hack, as all you do is simply add to the daytime look. Too easy! Follow these steps to get yourself glammed up at lightning speed and out of the door before you can say 'mince on toast'. Let's pick it up from Step 5 in the daytime look—I'm assuming you've already got your base make-up sorted. (Refer to the photo on page 189 if you need to for this look.)

Step 5:

ADD TO YOUR EYESHADOW TO CHANGE IT
UP FROM DAYTIME TO NIGHT-TIME.

Apply a base layer of eyeshadow as in Step 5 of the daytime look. Then, using an even darker eyeshadow palette than before (for an evening look, I prefer dark browns or golds), go over the crease of your eyelid, but this time bring the line slightly higher towards the brow and add more shading to the outside corner. Go over your lower lash line with the darker eyeshadow.

Step 6:

ADD SOME EYELINER.

To give definition to your eyes, apply a very thin line of eyeliner to the upper lash line; I use brown or black pencil eyeliner, but you can use pencil or liquid eyeliner—whatever you prefer. This takes some practice to get right, so have a cotton bud handy to tidy up any shaky lines!

Step 7:

MASCARA TIME!

Apply mascara to your lashes. Here, I've used **Maybelline The Colossal Big Shot** mascara, as it does amazing things for your lashes but also washes off easily. (I hate waterproof mascara, as it can seem to stay on like concrete.)

Step 8:

BLUSH TIME!

As for the daytime look, add your blush to the apples of your cheeks. I used **MAC Mineralize Blush** in Dainty again, but you could mix it up if you like.

Step 9:

FILL IN YOUR BROWS.

If you want, you can go for slightly more defined brows for an evening look, since your eyes will stand out more with the darker colours. Feel free to practise adding a bit more shape to your brows this time, rather than just filling in the bald spots.

Step 10:

APPLY COLOUR TO YOUR LIPS.

Here's where it gets fun! Lipstick shade options for getting glammed up are endless. For this look, I've used **MAC Lip Pencil** in Vino for the outline, and **Bobbi Brown Creamy Matte Lip Color** in Crushed Plum for the lip.

And that's it! Now you're one classy lazy girl.

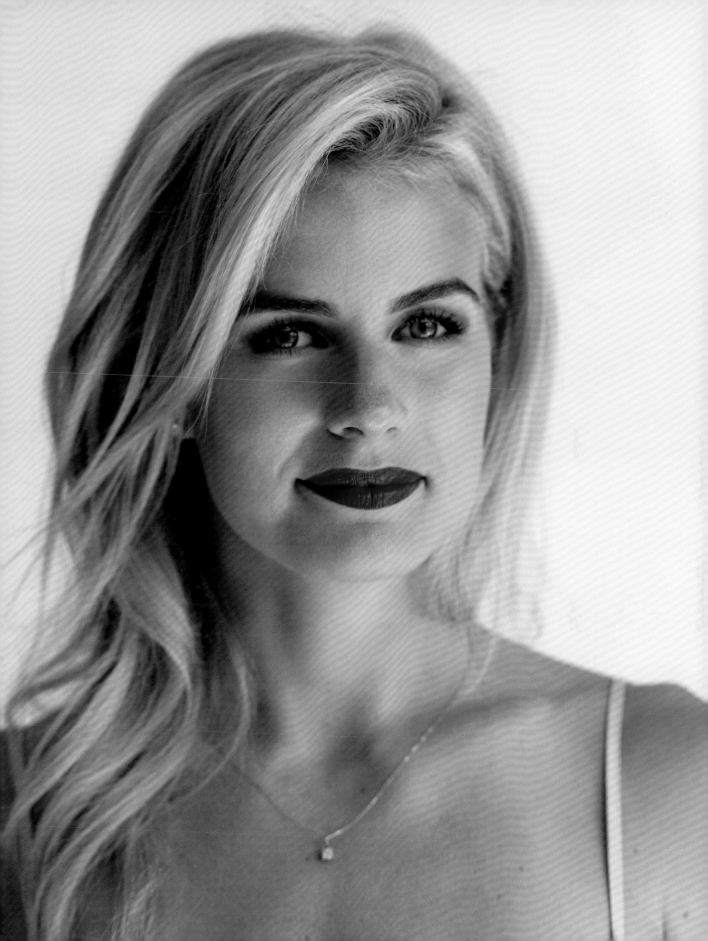

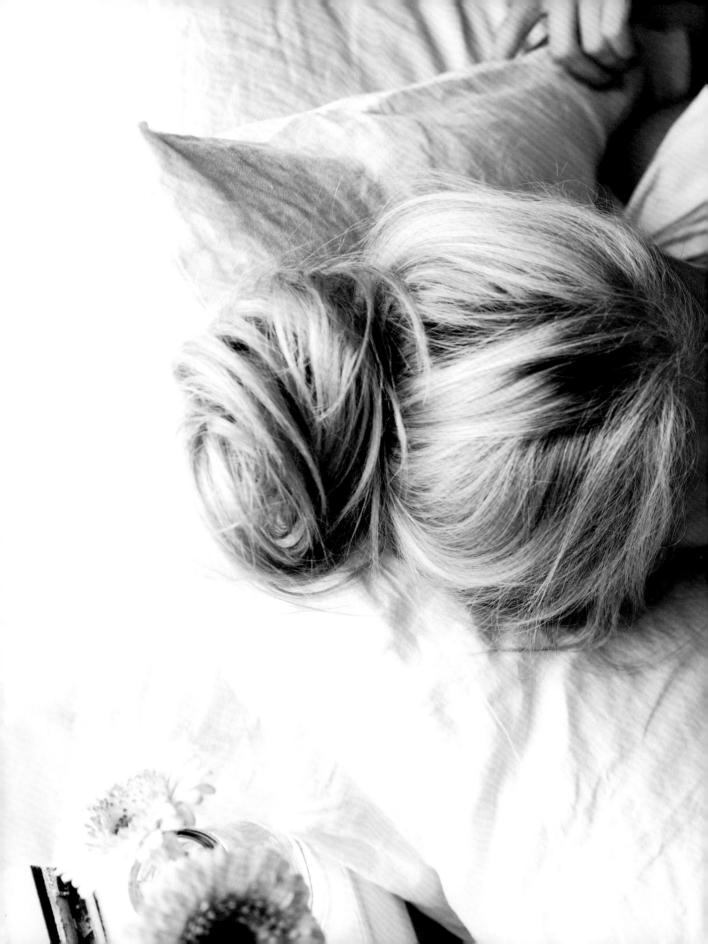

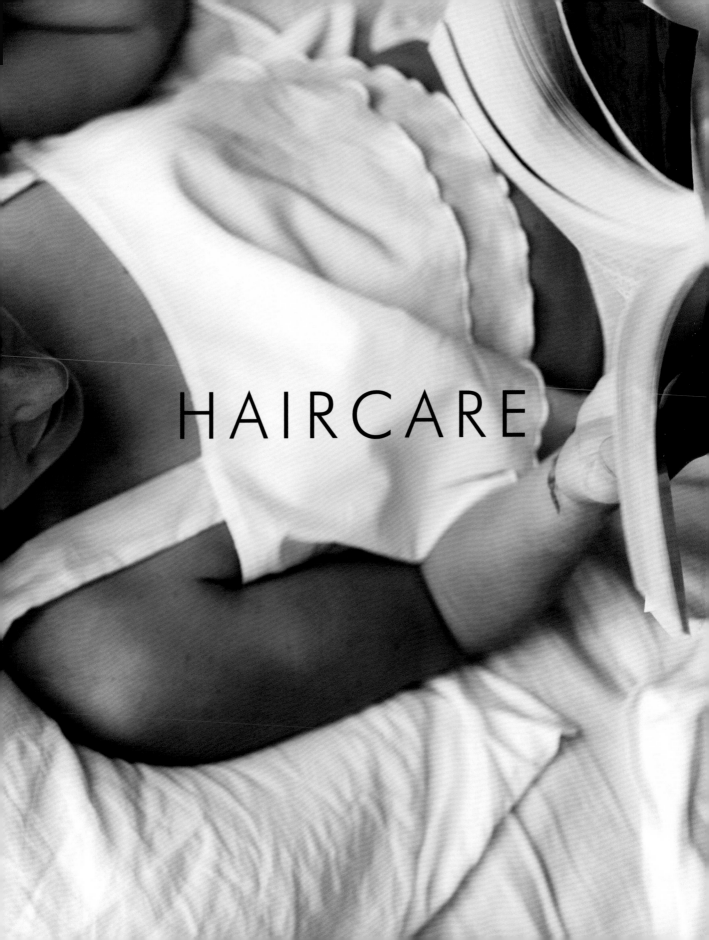

HAIRCARE

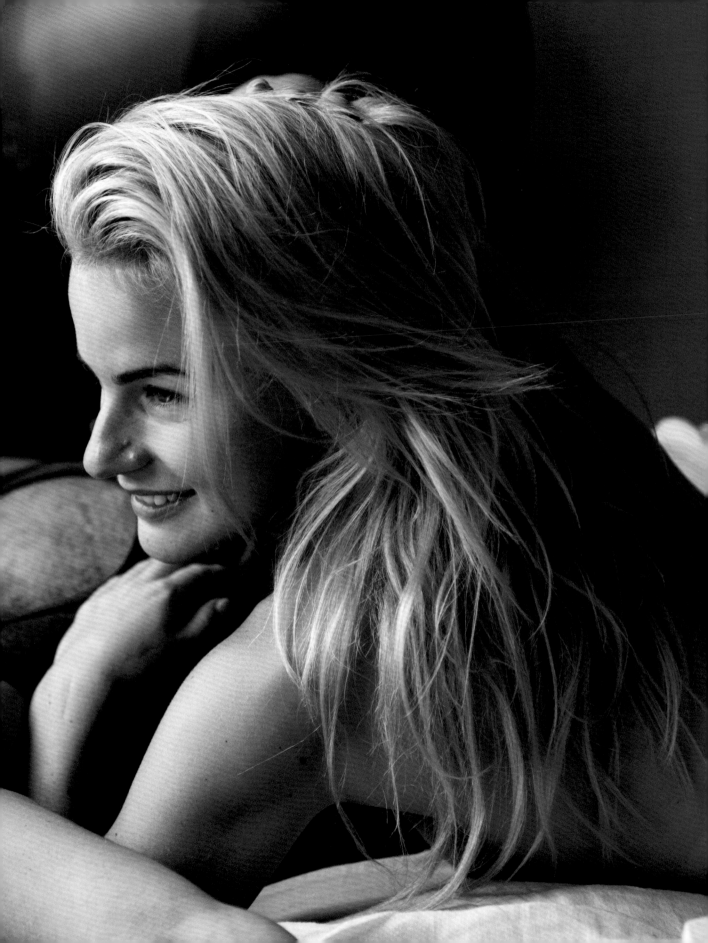

I'm pretty low-maintenance when it comes to doing my hair, but kind of the opposite when it comes to looking after it. I love having healthy hair, and I reckon that if you have healthy hair then it will look amazing no matter what you do to it.

I haven't always had healthy hair, though. When I was younger (circa the fake-tan stage), I dyed my hair from my natural blonde to dark brown. I used packet dye, and whenever my light regrowth began to appear I would just dye my whole head again. This meant I was dying my hair every few weeks, which was fine for a while . . . until I changed my mind and wanted to go back to blonde. Little did I know the journey I was embarking on! I had envisaged a quick trip to the salon, a few foils and I would be back to the blonde hair I'd had before. Not quite. It took a fair few trips to the salon (and a *very* ginger stage along the way) to finally achieve the blonde I wanted. And, even then, my poor hair was fried. It took almost a year for me to nurse it back to health, but the good news is that it did bounce back eventually.

Following are some of my tricks for keeping your hair healthy, shiny and gorgeous.

TOP TIPS FOR LUSTROUS LOCKS

1. Eat well

I know I've banged on about it in previous chapters, but I'll say it again just because I can: if you look after yourself on the inside it will show on the outside. Your hair is no exception. When you improve your diet, your hair improves too. Think beautiful and shiny!

2. Get your hair trimmed regularly

Even if you are trying to grow it out, get it trimmed. It will look ten times better, as it will stay healthy and not be full of split ends.

3. Try not to straighten your hair all the time

If you prefer straight hair, you can also smooth it with a hairdryer, which is a little less harsh on your hair than straighteners. Definitely still use a heat protector though (see my next tip).

4. Use products to protect your hair before you heat-style it

This could be a good heat-protecting spray and a nourishing oil, for example.

My haircare routine

I wash my hair every second day (or every third day at a stretch), and I prefer to use a **natural shampoo and conditioner** like the ecostore ones.

I like to use a little bit of **argan oil** on the ends of my hair every time I wash it, as it repairs the ends and gives it a lovely shine when I blow-dry it. Argan oil is produced from the kernels of the argan tree (there's a surprise), which is endemic to Morocco. You can actually use it in cooking as well as on your hair—and it's got a host of other beauty and health benefits, too. You can get it from most cosmetic and some health shops.

I also use a **volumising spray** before I blow-dry my hair to give it a bit of lift. I can't stand flat hair! I blow-dry my hair pretty much every time I wash it, as my hair doesn't really have any shape when it dries naturally. It's sort of curly in some areas and straight in others . . . which is why I tend to look a bit like a stray dog in summer time when I spend lots of time at the beach!

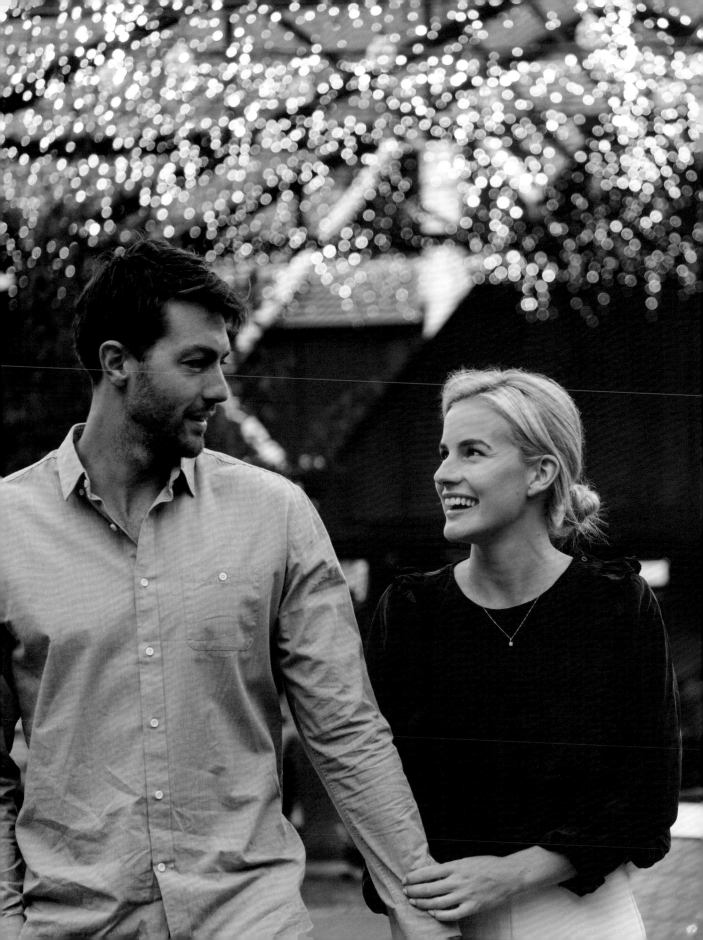

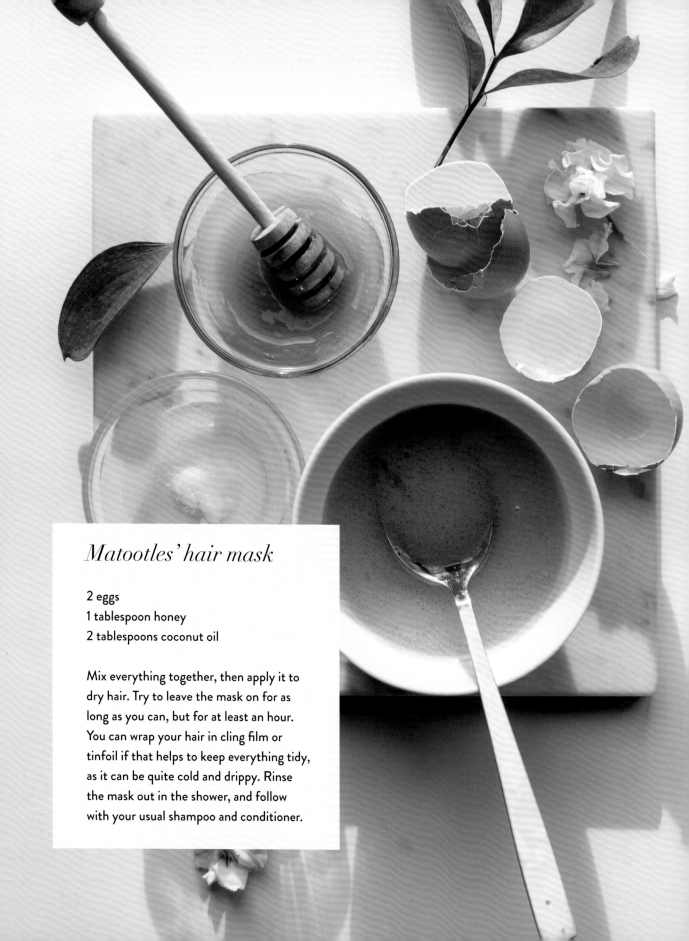

Matootles' hair mask

2 eggs
1 tablespoon honey
2 tablespoons coconut oil

Mix everything together, then apply it to
dry hair. Try to leave the mask on for as
long as you can, but for at least an hour.
You can wrap your hair in cling film or
tinfoil if that helps to keep everything tidy,
as it can be quite cold and drippy. Rinse
the mask out in the shower, and follow
with your usual shampoo and conditioner.

NOURISH YOUR HAIR

───────

Using a nourishing hair mask every week is really important to keep your hair feeling loved, and looking nice and shiny. I find a lot of hair masks are full of nasties, which I don't really like to leave on my scalp a long time, so I prefer to make my own (see page 196).

HOW TO PROPERLY
BLOW-DRY YOUR HAIR

───────

Now, this is not a classic lazy-girl manoeuvre. It takes far more time than the old 'put your head upside down and blow-dry all over' technique, but the results are totally worth it.

1. **Invest in a good hairdryer.** Don't go for one of those piddly travel ones; I'm talking a grunty professional dryer. I use an Elchim hairdryer and it's amazing! Try to get one with a high wattage—at least 1800—to prevent frizz. Also, if you're going to blow-dry your hair straight, you definitely need a nozzle attachment.

2. **Invest in a good hairbrush.** If you're looking for volume or a slight wave, then a round-barrel brush is what you want. The longer your hair, the bigger the barrel you will need. If you're wanting to blow-dry your hair straight, then a paddle brush is what you need.

3. **Prep your hair.** Pat your hair dry with a towel. *Don't* rub it; that creates frizz. Apply whatever products you like. If you're blowing curly hair straight, then use a straightening serum, but if you're trying to get volume then a volumising mousse or root spray will do the trick. I also recommend putting a little bit of argan oil through your hair too, to create some softness and shine, then comb through with a wide-tooth comb.

4. **Dry your hair all over until it is about 80 per cent dry.** You don't need the nozzle on for this part.

5. **Divide your hair into three sections: top, middle and bottom.** Tie or clip up the sections.
6. **Put the nozzle on your hairdryer, and start with the bottom section.** Wrap a 5 centimetre section of hair over your brush and hold it taught, then hold the dryer against the brush and gently pull down to brush your hair. Make sure you direct the airflow *down* the hair, from the roots to the ends.
7. **Repeat this section by section, until your whole head of hair is dry!**

Ta-da! I'm sure you now have beautiful, shiny hair . . . and hopefully your arm isn't too sore. It takes a *lot* of practice to master this, and everyone has a different way of styling their hair, but with time and practice you'll find your own special technique.

My go-to hairstyles

As I've said, I'm more about having healthy hair than I am about styling it, but there are definitely a few styles I favour during the day—mostly because they're easy!

♡ **A good old ponytail.** I'm a big fan of the ponytail, as it's super easy but can also be made to look really sleek for an evening look.

♡ **The messy bun.** If I'm on the third day of unwashed hair, it's pretty much a given that my hair will be in a messy bun. It's one of those 'I've made an effort to look like I haven't made an effort' looks—although this one also has to be paired with a good outfit, otherwise it just looks like you've just rolled out of bed.

♡ **Hair out.** I usually save this one for freshly washed and styled hair. I take a while to blow-dry my hair properly (I use a round brush and everything!), so I can't waste all that effort by putting it up.

♡ **If I'm off somewhere a bit flash . . .** If I'm going out to a special event, I'll either use hot rollers or pop into my local salon and let them get creative. Hot rollers are the best lazy-girl approach to a dressed-up look, as all you have to do is wait for them to heat up, roll them into sections of your hair, then get on with your life for an hour or so. Then take them out and BOOM! You are glam.

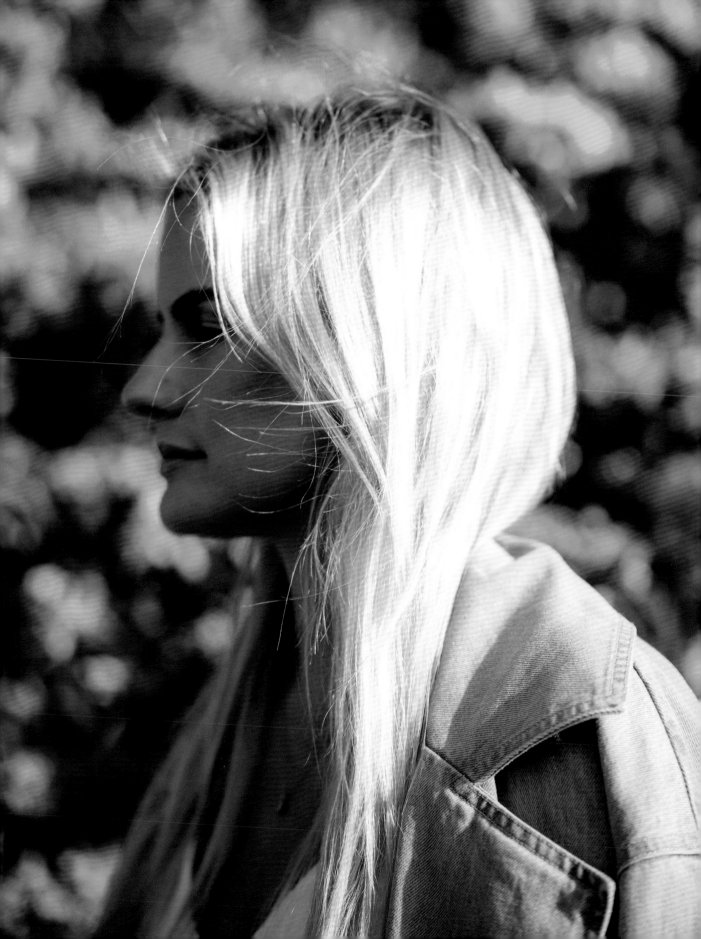

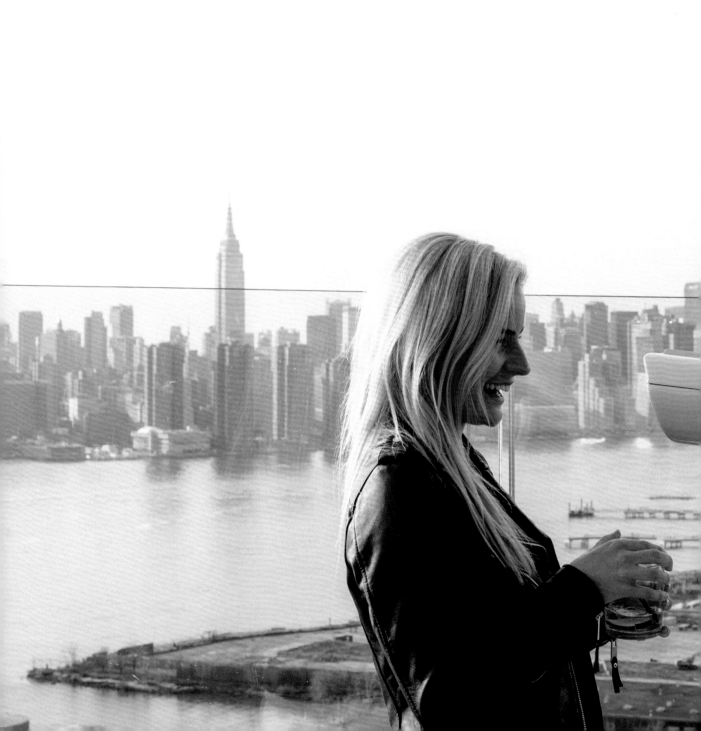

MY LIFE NOW

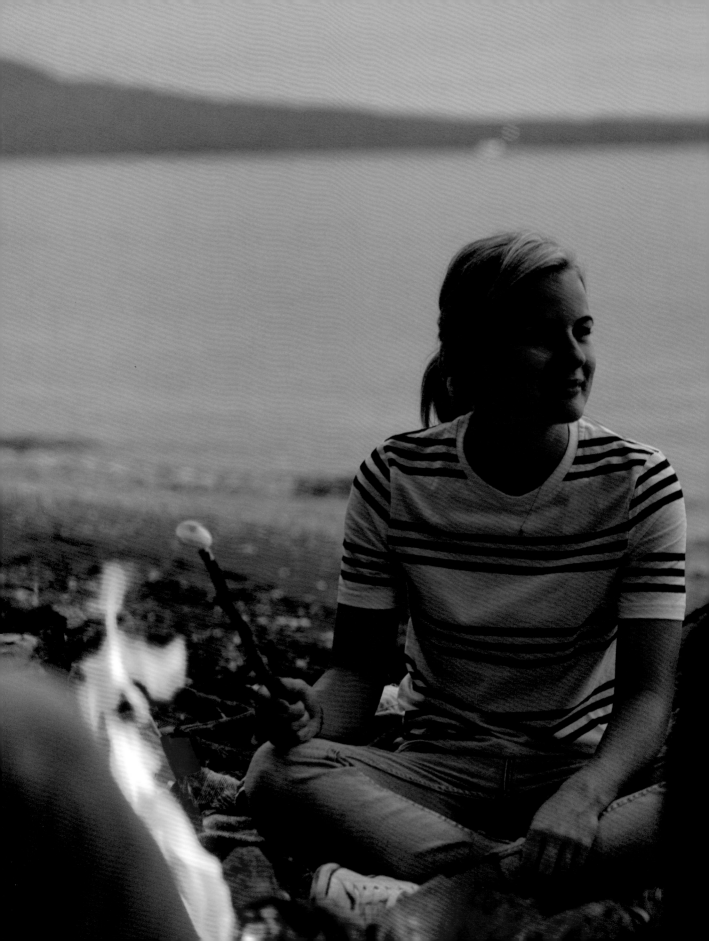

So, you've made it to the end of my book! (Or you got bored and skipped to the end. That's fine. I'm not offended . . . *sniff*.) I hope you've enjoyed my rambles, and that you've maybe even found one or two things that have been helpful or interesting along the way. I've designed this book to make it easy for you to dip in and out of whenever you need it, so I hope you'll come back to some of the things you found in its pages, too.

My goal with this book was to inspire those who read it (that's you!) to go out and live their best life, to look after themselves from the inside out, and to basically not worry about what other people think. Life is way too short to spend it worrying about what other people think of you. It's made for getting out there and *living* it, for spending with the people you love, and for doing the things that make you happy, fulfilled and feel great about yourself. Take risks, listen to your pals when they give you a reality check, and focus on living the best, most positive life you can.

I've made many mistakes in my life (some of which you now know about . . .), but I've tried to learn from them all. I wouldn't be who I am today without my mistakes, so in a way I'm grateful I made them (fake-tan and hair-dye mishaps and all). In this book, I wanted to share the things I've learned in life with you, so that you can learn from my mistakes too. Man, I wish 'future me' had given this book to 'past me'!

One of the things I really want to emphasise is that I actually do practise what I preach in this book. I'm not necessarily a health professional or a super-fit athlete; I'm just a very normal lazy girl, but if there's one thing I do know how to do it is love and respect myself. If you're not quite there yet, I really hope you get there, and that some of the things I've shared in these pages will help you to do that, because loving yourself is an incredible milestone to reach, and once you realise how much you are truly worth you will never look back.

Life is so much more fun when you feel good about yourself. Self-love isn't about being perfect (and this book isn't about you being like me); it's about learning who *you* are as a person, and what makes *you* special, and then accepting that for the awesome thing it is. We are all different, and that's what makes the world such an interesting place—if we were all the same it'd be pretty bloody boring, and I wouldn't even be writing this book.

Every single tip that I've provided in this book—whether it's how to live a more positive life, find your personal style, make deliciously easy and hearty food, or work out wherever and whenever you want—is something from my own life that I want to give to you. I want to share all the little tricks I've learned along the way so that you can get on the road to living your best life, even (and especially!) if you're a fellow lazy girl like me.

It is possible!

So go out, enjoy your life and. above all else, be happy.

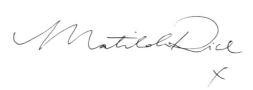

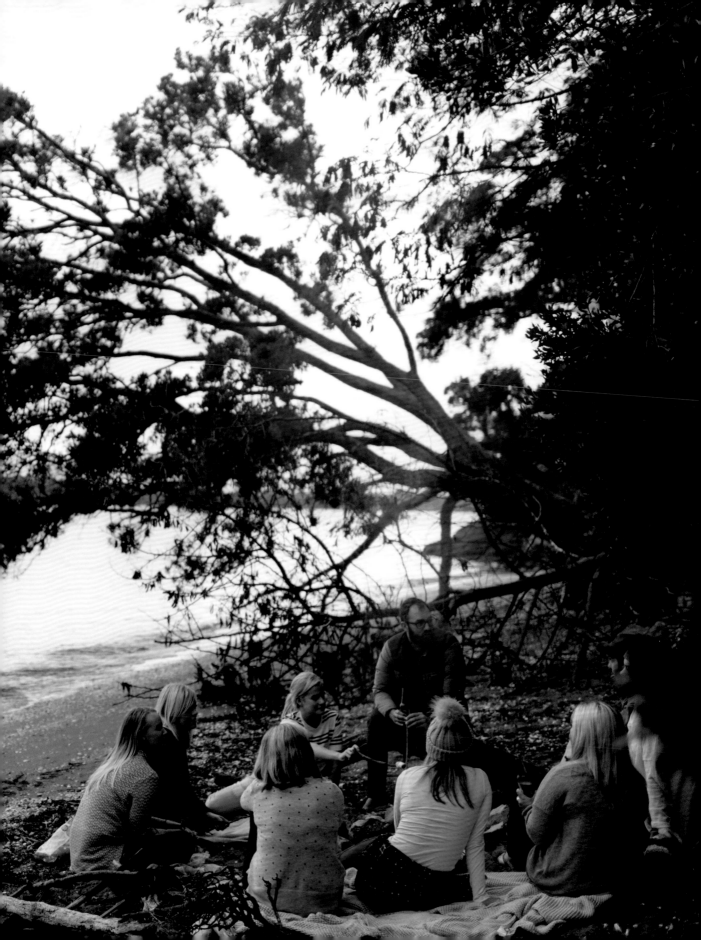

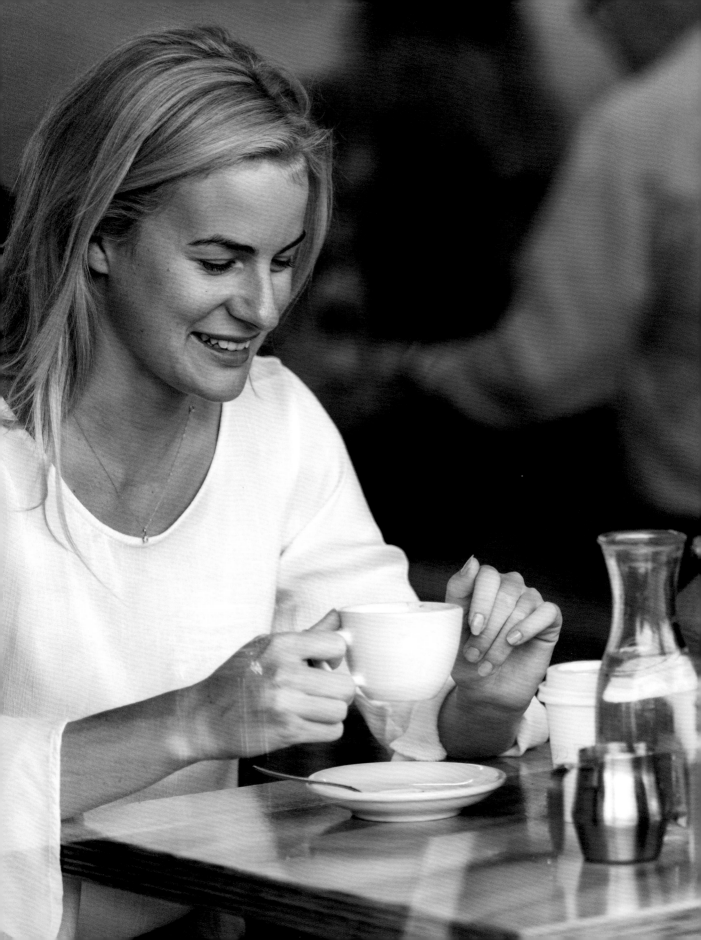

ACKNOWLEDGEMENTS

I am still pinching myself that this book has come to fruition, and am quite excited about adding 'author' to my Instagram bio. There are so many people who have contributed to the pages of this book, I don't know where to start!

First of all, thank you so much to Jenny Hellen and Kimberley Davis at Allen & Unwin for making it all happen and for being an absolute dream to work with, and to Kate Barraclough for making the pages come alive in the most stunning way. Thank you to Jo Bridgford, our amazing food stylist, for cooking and styling the recipes (they have never looked so good!). Obviously, there would be no book without them!

Thank you to my amazing family—Mum, Dad and Chloe—for constantly supporting me and loving me through all the different stages of my life.

To my darling Art, thank you for believing in me 100 per cent, and for patiently dealing with all the mood cycles that come with writing a book! Couldn't have done it without you.

Thank you to Jockey, Huffer and Ruby for dressing me, and to Zoe & Morgan for making me sparkle in your beautiful jewellery.

Last but not least, thank you so much to Emily Hlaváč Green for your incredible photography and creative skills, and for being a sounding board for all my ideas and a guinea pig for my workouts.

It really does take a village!

First published in 2017

Text copyright © Matilda Rice, 2017
Photography copyright © Emily Hlaváč-Green, 2017

Props for recipe photos kindly provided by
Delivision Food & Prop Styling, Citta Design,
Nest and Hayley Bridgford Ceramics

Allen & Unwin
Level 3, 228 Queen Street
Auckland 1010, New Zealand
Phone: (64 9) 377 3800

Email: info@allenandunwin.com
Web: www.allenandunwin.co.nz

83 Alexander Street
Crows Nest NSW 2065, Australia
Phone: (61 2) 8425 0100

A catalogue record for this book is available
from the National Library of New Zealand

ISBN 978 1 760631 51 2

Design by Kate Barraclough
Set in 10.5/15 pt Brandon Text
Printed and bound in China by
C&C Offset Printing Co., Ltd
10 9 8 7 6 5 4 3 2 1